JUST MANAGING: POWER AND CULTURE IN THE NATIONAL HEALTH SERVICE

ECONOMIC ISSUES IN HEALTH CARE

General editors

Professor Gavin Mooney
Health Economics Research Unit
Dept of Public Health
Medical School
Aberdeen AN9 2ZD

Dr Alistair McGuire
Dept of Sociological Studies
Wolfson College
University of Oxford
Oxford OX2 6UD

The Challenges of Medical Practice Variations
Edited by Tavs Folmer Andersen and Gavin Mooney (1990)

Private Exchange and Public Interest
By John Forbes (1990)

Rationing and Rationality in the National Health Service
Edited by Stephen J. Frankel and R. R. West (1993)

Just Managing – Power and Culture in the NHS
By Stephen Harrison, David J. Hunter, Gordon Marnoch
and Christopher Pollitt (1993)

Dental Care: An Economic View
By David Parkin and Brian Yule (1990)

JUST MANAGING

Power and Culture
in the
National Health Service

by

Stephen Harrison
David J. Hunter
Gordon Marnoch
and
Christopher Pollitt

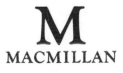

MACMILLAN

First published 1992 by
THE MACMILLAN PRESS LTD
Houndmills, Basingstoke, Hampshire RG21 2XS
and London
Companies and representatives
throughout the world

ISBN 0–333–51311–8 hardcover
ISBN 0–333–51312–6 paperback

A catalogue record for this book is available
from the British Library.

Printed and bound in Great Britain by
Mackays of Chatham PLC, Chatham, Kent.

Reprinted 1993

Contents

List of Tables

List of Abbreviations

BMA   British Medical Association
CHC   Community Health Council
CNO   Chief Nursing Officer
COHSE   Confederation of Health Service Employees
DHSS   Department of Health and Social Security
DGM   District General Manager
DHA   District Health Authority
DoH   Department of Health
FHSA   Family Health Services Authority
FPC   Family Practitioner Committee
GP   General (Medical) Practitioner
IPR   Individual Performance Review
NHS   National Health Service
MB   Management Budgeting
PI   Peformance Indicator
PRP   Performance Related Pay
RGM   Regional General Manager
RHA   Regional Health Authority
RAWP   Resource Allocation Working Party
RM   Resource Management
SHHD   Scottish Home and Health Department
UGM   Unit General Manager

Acknowledgements

The four of us have lived with the research on which this book is based for a long time. But even a team of four authors cannot produce a book alone. We have many to thank for their varying contributions to our efforts. Principally, they are: the Economic and Social Research Council for funding the research which we describe in Chapter 3; to Blackwell's for permission to reproduce material in a chapter which originally appeared in *Public Administration* 69 (1), Spring 1991 in an article which we wrote; all the respondents in our field sites in England and Scotland for their unfailing patience and generosity of time; Lin Clark and Nadia Davidson for tape transcripts of our interviews, and in Lin's case, for typing the manuscript of the book; and our 'counterfactual panel' (see Chapter 3) – Bob Nicholls, Alan Wilson, Stephen Griffin and Ian Johnston – who proffered helpful and frank advice throughout the research. Finally, we must thank the series editors – Alastair McGuire and Gavin Mooney – for their forbearance during the preparation of this book and for helpful comments on an earlier draft. We are, of course, responsible for the views and interpretations expressed and for any errors.

Introduction

For almost the whole of its existence, though more intensively in recent years, the British National Health Service (NHS) has been the subject of reorganisations and attempts to improve its management. But, the sceptics say, it makes no difference; the professionals and other health workers simply carry on in much the same way. These sceptical views can lead to two, very different, conclusions. One is that the attempts to improve management and organisation are a kind of froth (or even scum!) on the surface of an otherwise adequate service, which would do even better if its surface were skimmed. The other view is that the public ownership and near-monopoly status of the NHS form a fatal flaw in it, which no amount of improved organisation or management can effectively overcome. There are, of course, views in between these extremes.

As it happens, we do not subscribe to either extreme view, though our main concern in this book is not to assert our own views. Rather, we start from the observation that most of the organisational and managerial prescriptions which have under-pinned the changes to which we have referred have been insufficiently grounded in evidence; assertions and arguments about how the Service should be organised and managed have far exceeded the empirical base on which they ought to rest. The central purpose of this book is to provide an exposition and interpretation of the empirical evidence concerning the organisation and management of the NHS.

Although, in so doing, we review virtually all the published research evidence on the topic (there is not as much of it as we should like), the major thrust of our analysis is aimed at answering the question: what differences have the rather wide-ranging reforms, introduced after 1983 as a result of the Griffiths Report, made? Have the changes, as many of their proponents hoped and expected, led to major changes in the *culture* of the Service? Or have they, as some critics suggest simply been a diversion from more pressing issues of resourcing the Service? Or, as 'new right' critics argue, were the changes, unaccompanied by moves towards commercial competitive pressures, bound to result simply in further bureaucracy and 'empire-building'? Or is it that, as the Government might claim, everything is going to plan: some improvements have occurred and can be built upon in the introduction of yet more changes?

In attempting to shed light on these and other questions, we make use of research findings from our own earlier work and that of others from both before and after 1983. But the organisation and management of the Service are not static; even before some of the post-Griffiths studies to which we refer were published, the Government had produced the white paper *Working for Patients*, and thus embarked on a further large-scale reorganisation. A second main focus of our book, therefore, is to assess the implications and relevance of the research findings for the future NHS as projected in *Working for Patients* and its companion white papers *Promoting Better Health* and *Caring for People*.

The structure of our book is as follows. Chapter 1 is an introduction to the two concepts which appear in our title and which we use as key organising concepts throughout: *power*, and *culture*. As an adjunct to these, we also introduce the notion of *puzzlement* as an element in shaping the configuration of power and culture in a given context. Chapter 2 is a fairly straightforward summary of the main NHS managerial and organisational changes to which we referred above. Chapter 3 begins the summary of empirical material; its first half summarises research prior to the implementation of the Griffiths changes from 1984 onwards, whilst the second half summarises and contrasts the findings of our own major post-Griffiths study of 1987–8. We were, of course, not the only researchers to be interested in post-Griffiths NHS management, and Chapter 4 summarises the work of others and points to areas of convergence and divergence. Both Chapters 3 and 4 end by highlighting a number of puzzles, questions and inconsistencies between research findings. It is from the further exploration of such puzzles that better explanations often arise, and this is the purpose of Chapter 5: to provide an integrated and up-to-date account of our systematic empirical knowledge about organisation and management in the NHS. Finally, Chapter 6 carries this knowledge through into the post-white paper NHS.

By now the observant reader will be wondering what has all this got to do with *economics*, the subject matter of the series of which this volume forms part? We wish to suggest three crucial points at which the issues of economics and management connect in respect of the health service; our book sheds light on all of these, though we do not claim that it treats any of them exhaustively.

First, the impetus for managerial reform in the NHS during the 1980s comes very largely from perceived macroeconomic pressures. Increasing resource demands resulting from demographic pressures, new technological developments and rising hospitalisation rates have come up against macroeconomic policies which imply, on the contrary, a reduction in public expenditure. In the context of a service which constitutes the most popular sector of the British welfare state, the available policy options are few, and attempting *via* managerial and organisational reforms, to improve the efficiency of the NHS has been the chosen strategy.

Second, despite its rhetoric of rational decision making, management itself is rarely subject to microeconomic analysis; *investment* in better management, better systems and better information technology is treated as an act of faith. But there are significant opportunity costs to such investment. Whilst we are not ourselves competent to conduct such an analysis, and have not attempted to do so here, we do take the view that our study sheds some light on the scale and timing of the benefits that can be expected to flow from major structural change in a large and complex public service.

Third, the connection between economics and management has clearly become more important with the probable advent of competition in health care. The three white papers to which we referred above all contained proposals to introduce competition into primary health care, the hospital and community health services, and social care. We believe that our findings have important implications for the capacity of health care institutions to respond to such changes, and indeed to the desirability of their so doing.

Despite all this, our book is not, of course, primarily about economics, but about organisation and management.

STEVE HARRISON
DAVID J. HUNTER
Nuffield Institute for Health Services Studies, University of Leeds

GORDON MARNOCH
Department of Politics, University of Exeter

CHRISTOPHER POLLITT
Department of Government, Brunel University

CHAPTER 1

Power and Culture in the National Health Service

PREVIEW

The huge popularity of the NHS as a public institution has been matched, certainly during the last decade, by the enormity of the problems it has posed for the politicians responsible for it. Prime Ministers and Secretaries of State have wrestled with schemes for reorganising the Service, but at the time of writing it is brutally apparent that no generally accepted or well-tested solution has yet been found. In the following chapters we intend to explain why the NHS has proven so difficult to reform. We will focus not so much on 'high politics' as on the level where reform seems most frequently to come to grief – the month-by-month, year-by-year management of the Service. Our strategy will be to call on a very wide range of research (including some recent fieldwork of our own) in order to identify the congerie of practices, powers and perceptions which has shaped, and will continue to shape, the impact of governments' efforts to change the NHS.

The findings of researchers are varied, but we believe that certain important themes are clearly discernible. Government has sought increased control of the NHS, partly in order to promote efficiency and restrain the growth of public expenditure but partly, also, in an attempt to lessen discontents about different aspects of the Service. Our focus will be on hospitals rather than general practice or community care. In hospitals the government has had considerable success in installing, in the shape of general managers, a cadre of officials who are more responsive to central priorities than old style NHS administrators. General managers have been able to exercise considerable power, especially outside the specifically medical domain.

Nevertheless, alongside the real successes of general management there have also been less well-publicised disappointments. In our view these stem partly from the government's over simple prescription for the NHS's organisational ailments. During the 1980s the Conservative administration overestimated the extent to which the NHS could be managed according to private sector business models, and underestimated the power of doctors to resist challenges to their traditional way of doing things. Government may become increasingly able to insist on its policies in the face of resistance from the doctors' *national* representative bodies, but it has been the autonomy of doctors *locally* rather than the power of the British Medical Association which has blunted the drive for change.

Since 1989, however, the NHS has been facing a new upheaval, argu- ably more profound than anything which has gone before. In our final chapter we examine the prospects for management in the provider market heralded by *Working for Patients* (hereafter *WfP*). Clearly the white paper envisages further enhancement to the role of management. But will the medical profession go along? Will doctors be partners with managers or will they successfully resist managers, or will they seek, in larger numbers than hitherto, to take over management themselves? We argue that the provisions of *WfP*, taken as a whole, offer the skillful manager unprecedented opportunities for monitoring and shaping the behaviour of doctors. Managers will now have some of the tools in a way that they did not after the Griffiths Report of 1983. However, we also believe that many managers will find it extremely difficult to take advantage of these opportunities, not least because their agendas are likely to be overcrowded with a host of other priority issues. Costs and organisational changes are again likely to dominate the NHS manager's working week, with the quality of care and the effectiveness of medical practice continuing to take second or third place.

KEY CONCEPTS

Interpreting the changes of the last decade or so requires us to draw on over 40 research studies other than our own. These studies were not designed to be complementary to each other, so we have had to search for potentially unifying theories, themes or concepts which will allow us to marshall diversity within a single framework. The aim, of course, is to synthesise and clarify without seriously distorting the distinctiveness of the various studies. After some deliberation we chose *power*, including *puzzlement*, and *culture* as our key organising concepts.

Concepts are not free-floating entities; they relate to 'theories', that is, to particular sets of systematic perceptions about how the world (or some part of it such as organisations) 'works'. It should be noted that our discussion of theory is not merely an academic self-indulgence, since (implicitly more often than explicitly) theories underpin all purposeful action, in organisations as elsewhere in life. It follows that we have no real choice over whether to use theory or not; our only choice is to be implicit or explicit. We have chosen to be explicit, on the grounds that the reader will thereby be better able to judge our work. Implicit theorising can be dangerous – perhaps especially to those who pride themselves on their 'realism'. As J. M. Keynes once said, 'Practical men, who believe themselves to be quite exempt from any intellectual influences, are usually the slaves of some defunct economist' (Keynes, 1936).

We also freely confess that the *choice* of theory is not an entirely value- free choice. We do not mean by this that any old theory is as good as any other, but rather that one's perceptions of what issues are important (an outright value judgement) act back upon the relative appeal and usefulness of the different theories (for an extended discussion of values and theories, see Harrison, Hunter and Pollitt, 1990, Ch. 1.)

THEORIES OF ORGANISATION: POLITICAL PERSPECTIVES

The theory of organisations which we have adopted in this book is one which treats them as *political* systems (note the small 'p'). It is central to this perspective that individuals and groups within an organisation often have multiple and conflicting objectives and interests, and that their desire to defend these is an important determinant of behaviour. Where the interests of groups are in conflict, relative power is the major determinant of outcomes. This view of organisations has in recent years given rise to an increasing amount of academic literature (see, for instance, Dalton, 1959; Pfeffer, 1978; 1981; Pettigrew, 1973; Pollitt, 1990; Stephenson, 1985; Lee and Lawrence, 1985.) Of course, power is not all about conflict, whether covert or overt. The notion of *puzzlement* is important and should be introduced at this point. We return to it at greater length below but it is important to note that the issue of puzzlement and uncertainty should not be overlooked as a determining factor in much decision-making in which the play of power in conflict terms may not be present.

The reason for our choice of *power* as a key concept is thus obvious; it is a central component in the brand of theory that we are using. The basis of our choice of *culture* as our second key concept will not yet be so clear. Indeed, there are three reasons for the choice, the last of which is rather complex. Firstly, the notion of culture is probably the single most pervasive element in contemporary prescriptions for improving organisations; it was popularised in Peters and Waterman's *In Search of Excellence* (Peters and Waterman, 1982) and a succession of derivative works (see Meek, 1988 for a review). Secondly, as we noted in the Introduction, the concept surfaces in the stated aspirations of many of the proponents of recent organisational changes in the NHS (see, for instance, Institute of

Health Service Administrators, 1984, p. 69). 'Culture' is therefore relevant and topical.

The third reason is that culture (or rather, a particular conceptualisation of it) is also an integral part of our chosen theoretical approach. Culture denotes the prevailing assumptions and beliefs within a group; that which is 'taken for granted'. It is therefore an important indicator of what a group would be likely to perceive as legitimate and illegitimate, of change it might welcome and change it would more probably resist.

One last point about our theoretical position in general: we have not thought it necessary to discuss here the several definitions of 'organisation' itself that are available (for one discussion, see Pfeffer and Salancik, 1978, p. 245 ff.) But we do wish to make it clear that the micro-politics of the NHS with which we are concerned in this book are closely connected with its macro-politics (the subject of our earlier book *The Dynamics of British Health Policy*: Harrison, Hunter and Pollitt, 1990). Matters such as government policy are very much the everyday concern of many of the actors who populate the research studies that we summarise in later chapters.

Power

The concept of power has been developed over more than thirty years of academic writing, and has been the focus for a number of celebrated academic disputes. In a short introduction such as this, we cannot do justice to such a history, and have had to content ourselves with the essential definitions and clarifications, together with an account of just one dispute: that concerning the 'faces' or 'dimensions' of power.

Power is exercised when, as means of influence, the threat of a sanction is made (Dahl, 1976, p. 47); the sanction can, of course, be the withholding of a reward which would otherwise have been given (Bachrach and Baratz, 1970, p. 21). The logical corollary of power is, therefore, *dependence*; the two are inversely related (Pfeffer and Salancik, 1978, pp. 51–2). Freedom from dependence – from powerful influences – is usually termed *autonomy* (Dahl, 1976, p. 40). Since we are all somewhat dependent, in some way or other, autonomy is best conceived as a matter of degree rather than as an absolute state. A summary definition of what has been called the 'first face' or 'first dimension' of power is given by Bachrach and Baratz:

A power relationship exists when:

(a) there is a conflict over values or course of action between A and B;
(b) B complies with A's wishes; and
(c) B does so because he [*sic*] is fearful that A will deprive him of a

value or values which he regards more highly than those which would
have been achieved by noncompliance. (Bachrach and Baratz, 1970,
p. 24)

This approach to conceptualising power gives rise to two major difficulties, each of which has led to a further formulation. It should be
noted that these formulations are not alternatives to the 'first dimension'
definition given above, but are *additive* to it.

The first major difficulty arises from the obvious 'counterfactual'
problem; if we are researching power (or influence generally) how do
we know how B would have behaved had it not been for A's actions?
It may not be sufficient to ask B since self-respect may lead to a denial
of A's influence. The most cautious answer to this question is that of
Polsby (1980), who asserts that confident observations of an exercise of
power can *only* be made where overt conflict occurs, that is, where B is
seen to offer resistance which is subsequently overcome by A.

This, in turn, gives rise to the more fundamental criticism, first made
by Bachrach and Baratz (1962), that whilst such a view of power may
be adequate for the analysis of specific incidents, it is misleading when
applied across a whole polity (including, we would argue, an organisation or policy sector). This is because conclusions about the distribution
of power across the whole would rest solely upon the (presumably) small
minority of issues upon which overt conflict occurred. In other words,
such an analysis would have built into it the unwarranted assumption
that a virtual consensus existed on all matters which were not the subject
of such overt conflict.

In order to correct this perceived bias, Bachrach and Baratz proposed
to supplement the 'first face' conceptualisation with what they termed a
'second face' of power:

Power is also exercised when A devotes his [*sic*] energies to creating or
reinforcing social and political values and institutional practices that
limit that scope of the political process to public consideration of only
those issues which are comparatively innocuous to A. (Bachrach and
Baratz, 1970, p. 7)

If this seems somewhat abstract, the flavour of what Bachrach and Baratz
have in mind can be tasted by considering the kind of professional
strategies often employed in the NHS; how, for instance, has the clinical
freedom of doctors (a topic we treat at length in Chapter 2) remained
largely unchallenged (at least until recently)? This process of 'agenda-
structuring' is in principle observable, though it is not always related
to specific decisions or issues; a dominant group may control agendas in
such a way as to promote and protect its general dominance, even if not

consciously responding to a direct or potential challenge. A subordinate group or minority may decide not to 'make an issue' of something because they calculate that they are almost certain to be defeated (two aggrieved student nurses decide not to challenge a tyrannical ward sister or charge nurse). Thus the powerful remain powerful without having to act. Indeed, 'simply supporting the established political process tends to have this effect' (Bachrach and Baratz, 1970, p. 50).

The 'second face' of power has, in its turn, been criticised as inadequate (on its own) to analyse macro-level power distribution. Lukes posits, in addition, a 'third dimension' of power:

> [A] exercises power over [B] by influencing, shaping or determining his [sic] very wants. Indeed, is it not the supreme exercise of power to get another or others to have the desires you want them to have – that is to secure their compliance by controlling their thoughts and desires?   (Lukes, 1974, p. 23)

Lukes is here in effect raising the second of the two major difficulties for the first dimension of power, that is, its relationship to *authority*. Although writers have disagreed as to whether or not authority is a sub-category of the first dimension of power (cf. Dahl, 1976, p. 60; Bachrach and Baratz, 1970, p. 32), they do agree that authority involves legitimacy; B is more likely to comply with A's desires where B considers A and/or his or her desires to be legitimate, that is, authoritative. In this formulation, authority lies in B's perceptions, rather than being, as often treated, an attribute of formal organisation structures.

It is an obvious strategy, therefore, for A to try to enhance his or her authority; 'leaders in a political system try to convert their influence into authority' (Dahl, 1976, p. 60). Though the connection is rarely made, precisely the same line of reasoning underpins the contemporary literature (to which we referred above) on managing organisational cultures. All other things being equal, the management pronouncements of a 'caring', humanistic culture may be regarded by employees as more legitimate than that of a 'gradgrind' management. We shall return to this in the next section.

The standard objection to Lukes's position is that since by definition, the third dimension of power involves B's values and preferences being shaped by A, there remain no observable conflicts of values and therefore no observable exercise of power. Lukes himself defends his position by arguing that it is valid for an observer to make a judgement about the 'real' ('objective') interests of actors: to reach, for instance, a conclusion that B has been manipulated into adopting preferences which are actually against B's interests (Lukes, 1974, ch. 8). Whilst this argument is probably valid, it requires, as Lukes himself makes clear, careful and disciplined usage. But the problem of observation would be much reduced if A were actually to admit what was going on: if attempts to shape B's values and preferences were acknowledged to be such. As we shall see, this may often be the case with attempts to modify organisational culture.

Before moving on to the issue of *puzzlement* and the concept of culture we need to take note of two further complications in the study of power. These are, first, the problem of *collective action* and, second, the possibility of *luck* (as opposed to power) helping to determine outcomes.

The problem with collective action is that a potential opposition may not act *because of its own difficulties in organising* rather than because it is being restrained or directly attacked by a dominant group. Thus a large majority of UK citizens may favour increased spending on the NHS yet still find it difficult to organise an effective campaign. Though they all disagree with the government's restrictions on spending they also disagree among themselves as to what should be done instead. Some want to spend more on heart surgery, some on care for the elderly, some on maternity services or family planning. Some favour Parliamentary lobbying, others strikes, yet others a media campaign. They may be unable to 'get their act together', to organise as a single unit and fight for a single, alternative policy to the government's. Thus there is no 'campaign' and little conflict – the government doesn't have to exert *either* first or second face power because the potential opposition is itself ineffective (Olsen, 1971; Dowding, forthcoming).

Finally, that some are strong and others weak may be a question of luck rather than power. Britain's economy was considerably strengthened during the 1970s and '80s by the flows of oil and gas from the North Sea. But the existence of these natural assets was itself a matter of luck rather than some exercise of power. In the health field power/dependency relationships were altered by both the advent of AIDS and the high proportionate growth of the elderly section of the population. These may have put some health care groups in stronger (or weaker) bargaining positions, but it would be misleading to assume that this increase (decrease) in their power was itself the result of a 'power play'. They were simply lucky (unlucky).

Puzzlement

Politics is not all about conflict and power. Puzzlement and uncertainty are common features in respect of policy-making and implementation. It is a blinkered view of politics to believe that it is only present where there is disagreement about who gets what, when and how. As Heclo (1975, p. 305) succinctly puts it: 'politics finds its sources not only in power but also in uncertainty – men [sic] collectively

wondering what to do'. Governments, and those employed by or working for them or their agencies, not only indulge in power-play or
power; they also puzzle. Heclo again: 'policy-making is a form of
collective puzzlement on society's behalf; it entails both deciding and
knowing'. A pure power approach is insufficient to explain all the
outputs from the 'black box' we call policy. In the NHS, the assault of
managerialism on health is viewed in confrontational terms as posing
a direct challenge to the medical profession's interests. It is held up
as a good example of the interplay of conflict and power. But the
growth of managerialism can also be interpreted as a response to
the increasingly complex issues which beset all developed health care
systems and therefore confront policy-makers with difficult choices.
The issues include problems of rationing care – a feature of all systems but no less easy to resolve for all that; of determing the optimal levels of spending on health services; and of obtaining robust
information on the impact of medical interventions on health status.

This is not to suggest that the doctor-manager relationship and the
power dimension permeating it is of no consequence. But it may not be
the only trigger governing change or the perceived need to do something.
When puzzlement and uncertainty are present in policy-making and also
implementation, managerialism has considerable appeal because of its
association with rational problem-solving, a focus on actions, change
and 'getting things done', and on systematic analysis based on sound
information.

The contribution of the 'health problem' to puzzlement and uncertainty
cannot be overstated. The problem stems from a series of fundamental
uncertainties (Thompson, 1981). For a start, the health status of a population as well as the means for improving it remain cloudy (Mooney and
Loft, 1989). It is not necessary to travel far down the road of trying to
discover answers to these puzzles before quickly becoming embroiled in
the complexities involved in assessing whether greater public investment
in health actually produces a healthier population. As Mooney and Loft
argue

> medical decision-making attempts, *inter alia*, to analyse the often
> difficult relationship between certain types of health care inputs (for
> example, those comparing certain treatment regimes) and certain
> types of health outputs – and in a world of uncertainty. How this
> is actually done is itself shrouded in uncertainty or more accurately
> ignorance. (1989, p. 21)

Puzzlement and uncertainty represent one set of explanations underpin-
ning Lipsky's (1980) theory of 'street-level bureaucracy'. Those embraced
by the terms are the employees of a wide range of public services –

schools, hospitals, police, housing, courts and so on – who act with, and have wide discretion over, the dispensation of services and allocation of resources. Street-level bureaucrats are major recipients of public resources. Users of services invariably experience government through them, and their actions often *are* the policies provided by government as a result of the substantial discretion allowed them in the execution of their work. In addition, they enjoy relative autonomy from organisational authority. Attempts to curtail this are viewed as illegitimate and constitute grounds for non-compliance. Street-level bureaucrats *expect*, by virtue of their position, themselves to make initial decisions about access to services or whatever. In this, they make a distinction between their interests as professionals from those of managers.

Doctors represent a key group of street-level bureaucrats in part because a chief characteristic of their work is the conflicting and ambiguous nature of its goals. For example, is the goal of the NHS to deal with ill-health or promote health? Very different strategies are implied by each. Moreover, many goals are articulated at an idealised level of abstraction which makes their achievement problematic. Of course, the goals may be ambiguous and/or abstract in order to bury conflicts or, at any rate, to ensure they remain latent. Hence, the concept of power may be responsible for, or at least be a contributory factor to, the ambiguity. But it is also plausible to argue that a major source of ambiguity lies in puzzlement or in what Lipsky calls 'social service technologies' (*ibid.*, p. 41). Accordingly

> when there are uncertainties over what will or will not work, there is greater room for admitting and tolerating a variety of approaches and objectives. In such an intention there is often a hunger for discovering successful techniques . . .

Perhaps the quest for managerial control in the NHS is an attempt by policy-makers to sate their appetite–at least for the time being.

Organisational Culture

The notion of organisational culture has its intellectual roots in sociology and anthropology. Recently, however, it has been widely applied to the field of organisation and management studies. It is important to note that although there are at least two schools of writing about culture, only one of these has been to any great extent transported into management texts about organisational culture. This approach defines culture rather broadly as the total body of material artefacts, ideas, beliefs and behaviours which are transmitted from generation to generation within a polity; as Meek (1988, p. 453) puts it, 'all that is human within the organisation'. It also treats culture in rather a functional way: culture is something which an organisation 'has', and which may be deliberately manipulated in order to produce certain effects (Cameron and Ettington, 1988). As noted above, the most prominent work in this genre is Peters and Waterman's *In Search of Excellence* (Peters and Waterman, 1982). In this book the authors conclude that successful organisations were characterised by a dominant and homogeneous culture:

> Without exception, the dominance and coherence of culture proved to be an essential quality of the excellent companies. Moreover, the stronger the culture and the more it was directed toward the marketplace, the less need was there for policy manuals, organisation charts, or detailed procedures and rules. In these companies, people way down the line know what they are supposed to do in most situations because the handful of guiding values is crystal clear.   (Peters and Waterman, 1982, pp. 75–6)

Peters and Waterman go on to describe a number of ways in which such an organisational culture can be constructed; their emphasis is very much on the approach adopted by top managers in acting as role models, propagating organisational 'myths' which reinforce managerial legitimacy, and so on (p. 287 ff). There are, of course, at least two kinds of objection to this approach. One, which we shall not be concerned with further, is ethical; it can be argued that, along with all conscious exercises of the third dimension of power, people are being manipulated in a manner reminiscent of 'Big Brother'. Organisational members who fail to be thus manipulated will be perceived as deviant (Meek, 1988) and therefore be subjected to 'first dimension' sanctions.

The second objection is that organisations may well not exhibit homogeneous cultures and that it may be much more difficult than Peters and Waterman suggest deliberately to produce such a culture (Feldman, 1986). We referred above to two schools of writing on the topic but have so far looked at only one. The second school meets the objections that we have raised, for it is less embracing; it treats culture as an 'ideational system' (Allaire and Firsirotu, 1984) only, allowing for the possibility that beliefs and behaviours may diverge (Bate, 1984). This more anthropological perspective conceives an organisation's culture as something the organisation *is* rather than something it *has*. It also recognises the possibility that several different cultures may coexist within an organisation (Meek, 1988). Since it is precisely at times of change that divergence between beliefs and behaviours may occur (Allaire and Firsirotu, 1984) we are naturally drawn to this second approach. We therefore employ the notion of organisational culture to signify the systems of values, beliefs and ideas held by groups within the organisation; amongst the questions that we shall be asking of the research findings which we summarise in later chapters are: how homogeneous is the NHS culture? What differences are there between professional and other groups? Do differences conflict or complement each other? What changes have taken place, and how deep have they gone? Have they transformed deep cultural assumptions and beliefs or merely shifted the 'climate' of surface attitudes?

A number of authorities have proposed systems for classifying cultural change (e.g. Bate, 1984; Cameron and Ettington, 1988; Gagliardi, 1986; Feldman, 1986). One that has proved particularly popular in the UK is that developed over a number of years by Charles Handy (Handy, 1976; 1985). Handy offers a loose but vivid characterisation of four very different cultures, and we will borrow from his typology later in this book. He recognises that actual organisations and sub-organisations may display mixtures of his four 'ideal types', and that different parts of the same organisation may exhibit strongly contrasting sub-cultures (e.g. as between the production and marketing divisions of a manufacturing company).

Handy's first cultural type is the *power culture*. It is characterised by an assumption that strong, charismatic, central leadership is the most appropriate organisational form. Committee structures and formal rules are believed to be less important than the personality of the leader and the need for a dynamic response to opportunities for growth and dominance. Since these have never seemed to be particularly prominent features of the NHS culture we will not say much more about this type.

The NHS has, however, been likened to Handy's second type, the *role culture*. Here the basic assumption is that the organisation will proceed through the making and adjustment of a complex set of rules. Authority will be carefully subdivided between different specialist groups or functions. Thus job descriptions will frequently be regarded as more important than the individuals who fill those jobs. Jobs will be carefully ranked in hierarchies so that the common assumption will be that uncertainties are resolved by referring them 'up' for authoritative resolution. Bureaucratic rationality is seen as the normal and legitimate way of doing things (Handy, 1976, p. 179–90). Procedural correctness is held to be very important and dynamic, stylish action, instead of being regarded as praiseworthy (power culture), is usually considered disruptive and inappropriate.

By contrast, the prime emphasis in the *task culture* is on achieving results by the application of relevant expertise. Influence is based on expertise rather than on the kind of positional authority which dominates in role cultures. Hierarchies may be regarded as rather cumbersome and ineffective – instead the task culture spawns team- or matrix-working. The attitude is one of 'Let's get together the people who really know about this issue and give them freedom to produce an effective solution – whatever their titles or specialisms'. Task cultures can be difficult to discipline because of their creativity and resistance to central regulation. However, they can achieve high productivity, especially in an environment of opportunity and growth.

Finally, Handy describes a *person culture* in which the creative individual is the centre of attention and admiration. If there is a formal structure to the organisation 'it exists only to serve and assist the individuals within it' (Handy, 1976, p. 183). The organisation is focussed on a cluster of individual stars, and the local myths and rituals are woven around the idiosyncracies of these personalities. Handy suggests that some architects' partnerships or barristers' chambers approach this model – we might add that so do some consultants' firms. The medical profession has been clever enough to have created little cells of personal culture within a larger role culture. NHS administrators, nurses and paramedical staff operate in well-defined hierarchies with an abundance of rules and regulations, but the consultant body has hitherto worked within an exceedingly vague job description and has sported its fair share of prima donnas. Table 1.1 summarises some of those key features of Handy's typology.

Handy believes there to be an important relationship between the cultural type and the effectiveness of the organisation. He does *not* suggest that there is one best culture, but rather argues that effectiveness comes from the development of a culture which 'fits' the environmental and strategic contingencies facing the organisation. Thus, for example, if the environment is fairly stable, resources fairly tight, and the requirement is for high volume but essentially routine operations, then a role culture will fit well. If the environment is changing more rapidly (e.g. through technological advances) and resources are reasonably plentiful, then a more flexible, results-oriented system of beliefs and assumptions will serve the organisation well, and the task culture will probably outperform a more slow-moving role culture.

In his later work Handy developed the theory that a cultural crisis had begun to affect many of the large bureaucratic organisations which, by the 1970s, had come to dominate our society, both in the public and the private sectors (Handy, 1985). He saw a developing tension between the bureaucratic impulse towards greater uniformity and size and the demands of a more affluent and educated society for more choice and personal expression. The latter pressures impacted on organisations both through the demands of customers/clients and through the aspirations of their own employees for jobs which allowed for more creativity and flexibility. The tension was beginning to be resolved by the emergence

Table 1.1 Summary of power relations within Handy's four cultural types

Cultural 'Ideal Type'	Location of dominant power
Power	One or a few key individuals at the centre of the organisational web. They need to be dynamic, risk-taking etc. if the organisation is to adapt to a changing environment.
Role	Power and authority largely coterminous. Authority is parcelled out in well-defined units to particular positions in the hierarchy. Those in the top positions hold the largest amounts. Expert power is accepted, but only in its allotted place ('on tap but not on top').
Task	Power lies with those who are positioned at the intersections of networks of specialist, task-oriented groups. These may be experts, or simply good 'fixers'. In general power is more widely dispersed than in any of the other three types. It is a team culture in which the skills of collective organising are highly valued.
Person	Power lies with the 'star' individuals around whom the organisation is formed. The power base is usually expertise of some kind, so neither the 'fixers' of the task culture nor the entrepreneurs or 'dictators' of the power culture will be prominent here. Rules are few and controls are light. Collective action occurs only when there is mutual agreement between the 'stars'.

of a new type of organisation, a cultural hybrid in which the role culture was considerably modified by the growth of strong elements of task and even person cultures. This cultural hybrid would be characterised by:

• High autonomy for each part of the organisation (e.g. the ward or primary care team). The centre will hold each part accountable for certain key achievements, but will not attempt to prescribe in detail how these objectives are to be met.
• Staff enjoy higher personal involvement and commitment because they now identify more with their local, semi-autonomous unit than with the huge, impersonal totality of the organisation.
• An expert professional core, with elements of person culture-type freedoms.
• Many staff outside this core would be employed on short term contracts. Again, these would specify results and quality standards with some precision, but would be much less prescriptive about methods.
• A much slimmed-down middle management. The combination of improved information technologies with a more results-oriented, contract based approach would reduce the need for the rule-making, controlling administrators so characteristic of role cultures. The remaining

managers would be more concerned with strategic issues and contract compliance.

Interestingly, Handy chooses the hospital as an example of such a new hybrid, federally-structured organisation. And, as we shall see, some elements of this kind of thinking seem to have coloured the proposals in *Working for Patients*.

We have considerable reservations about Handy's vision of the future – on grounds both of the accuracy of his prediction and the desirability of some of its elements. For example, we are not as sanguine as he appears to be that the influence of management will decline relative to expert professional groups. Neither are we comfortable with the implications of a larger and larger proportion of the workforce being employed mainly or exclusively on short term contracts. Nevertheless, we recognise that during the second half of the 1980s this and similar visions have acquired great ideological and practical influence. There is a confusion of terms and labels around this emergent new model. Some writers stress its cultural dimension while others concentrate on associated organisational techniques and management behaviours. We need to deal with both, and have therefore chosen a fairly broad term to describe this bundle of assumptions and arrangements – the *post-Fordist model*.

POWER AND CULTURE: FORDISM AND POST-FORDISM

A daunting mass of literature (some of it fairly impenetrable) has sprung up around the post-Fordist model (see, for a popular example, Mulgen, 1988, or for more detailed/academic treatments, Lipietz, 1987 or Hoggett, 1990). It is not our intention to go far into that here. Rather we wish to deploy the post-Fordist model as a loose organising device which enables us to pigeonhole certain sets of ideas and practices about the management of the NHS. It enables us to distinguish between two alternative and to some degree contradictory responses to the problems which the NHS has posed for government. The first, 'Fordist', response has been to try to tighten direct controls – to measure, to regulate, to strengthen line management, to collect more and more detailed data and to insist, from 'the top', that the data are formatted in a uniform, centrally-defined way. This is essentially a 'command' approach. It carries a strong flavour of the school of management associated with F. W. Taylor. It is also a bureaucratic response which comes naturally from an organisation with a predominantly role-type culture. At its core is the notion that management needs to control the workforce by specifying in some detail what is to be done, how it is to be done, and in what quantity it is to be done. It is a mass production approach, oriented to efficiency and predictability. During the late 1970s and 1980s this way of thinking was increasingly applied to the UK public services sector, including the NHS (Pollitt, 1990a).

By contrast a post-Fordist response would be to fragment the organization and leave each constituent part or unit to deal with the detailed problems of resource allocation, methods of work, organisation charts and so on. If these came to differ extensively from one unit to the next, so be it. At the centre, top management would be left with the strategic tasks only. Its main concerns would include the setting of overall outcome targets, quality standards and global budgets. Relations between the centre and the constituent units would be mainly contractual – those units which failed to meet their targets would suffer well-defined penalties and would have to reform themselves or, eventually, disappear. Survival would go to the fittest, and the fittest would be those who developed flexible internal structures and procedures which enabled them to respond quickly and effectively to the latest changes in market demands and/or strategic targets. The appropriate culture for such units would presumably be nearer Handy's task type than his role type, though the latter might persist in those local environments where the demands on the organisation were stable and predictable.

How, then, do power and culture connect, one with the other? The answer must be that the connections are intimate and subtle. On the first dimension of power, culture is an obvious resource. Whichever actors in a conflict can claim to have the prevailing culture on their side can thereby strengthen their position. So in a role culture, for example, the innovative nurse who tries at a meeting to take open issue with consultant's way of doing things is at an immediate disadvantage – more so than in a task culture, where, if the subordinate can claim some expertise, s/he is more likely to get a fair hearing, irrespective of nominal rank.

Equally, the prevailing culture can also influence the second face of power. Far from winning the argument at the meeting our innovative nurse, in a strict role culture, may not even be able to get the issue (whatever it may be) onto the agenda. The whole idea of someone of junior status proposing an agenda item may effectively be ruled out.

It is in relation to the third dimension of power, however, that cultural factors perhaps have their most subtle influence. For cultural assumptions, symbols and rituals may focus attention on certain aspects of the work process and draw it away from others. Certain issues are highlighted and others backgrounded. It may not even *occur* to our imagined nurse that there is an issue to be raised, a problem to be addressed. If the culture is one where subordinates are not *expected* to have new ideas, they may not expend much energy thinking of them – it becomes a pointless activity.

Table 1.2   The shift to post-Fordism

Fordist or 'Command' model of Management	*Post-Fordist Model*
1. *Culture.* Role/bureaucratic	1. *Culture.* Hybrid of task and role with elements of person culture.
2. *Typical organisational structure.* Hierarchy; 'integrated firm', centralised.	2. *Typical organisational structure.* Network of specialised and/or local units held together by contractual relationships, within the broad framework of a strategic plan. Decentralised.
3. *Dominant criterion for action.* Conformance to rules and procedures.	3. *Dominant criterion for action.* Achieving results.
4. *Style of production or service delivery.* Mass production. Infequent design changes. Producer-driven.	4. *Style of production or service delivery.* Small batch or individually-tailored production. Frequent design changes. Consumer-responsive.
5. *Typical employee status.* Permanent, career employees.	5. *Typical employee status.* Small core of permanent professionals, larger number of staff on a variety of types of whole time or part time term contracts.
6. *Key management tasks.* Fix effort levels. Specify work methods. Ensure employee compliance.	6. *Key management tasks.* Develop employee commitment. Ensure output targets are met. Sustain close relationships with other units and with the centre.

The much-vaunted transition from Fordist to post-Fordist models of management has somewhat contradictory implications for the power/culture interface (see Table 1.2). On the one hand it is frequently portrayed as a liberating force for the employee. The dead hand of bureaucracy will be removed. Innovation will be encouraged. Flexibility will be at a premium. Performance will be rewarded. The appropriate culture for such an organisation will surely be open, positive, valuing of staff creativity and productivity.

Yet there is a dark side to post-Fordism. A number of writers have pointed out that post-Fordist 'human resource management' requires from employees not merely the compliance of the old Fordist, bureaucratic regimes, but positive commitment and enthusiasm (Storey, 1989). This is the key to several characteristic post-Fordist devices, such as quality circles or merit pay. The nine-to-five mentality is no longer enough: staff are now expected to 'go the extra mile', and not to gripe about union rules or late homecomings. In so far as top management believes it can now re-fashion organisational cultures (a belief we question later in this volume) it may do so in a way which erodes employee protections and punishes the doubting and disaffected. The vision of NHS staff rising early to gather and sing the hospital song before tramping happily off to work is not a wholly reassuring one.

DOCTOR POWER

Although this is a book about NHS management it will surprise few readers that the medical profession looms large in its pages. As already indicated, research shows that doctor power has frequently proven more than a match for manager power. It may be helpful, therefore, to conclude this chapter with a brief examination of the nature of medical power. The issue is returned to in Chapter 5.

In our view doctor power can usefully be thought of as having two substantially distinct components. On one level doctors constitute a powerful pressure group. Their national 'peak' associations – the British Medical Association and the Royal Colleges – are well organised and well-resourced, and long ago secured the right to be consulted about all manner of proposed government changes to the NHS (Haywood and Hunter, 1982). Following the creation of the NHS in 1948 this relationship became a particularly intimate one, and political theorists frequently cite it as an example of 'meso-corporatism' (Cawson, 1985). For our purposes we refer to this component of doctor power as 'macropower'. Its origins lie with the original, nineteenth century bargain between the state and the doctors in which the former secured monopoly professional status in return for a commitment to maintain standards, control members and in other ways relieve the state of the burden of regulating the rapidly growing field of organised medicine. As health care services have become more complex still, and the number of occupational groups involved has multiplied, the dominance of the medical profession may have been slightly diluted, but its macropower has remained considerable (Haywood and Hunter, 1982).

But if doctors are powerful collectively at national level, they are also powerful individually at a local level. They control the admission and discharge of patients, the diagnosis of those patients' conditions and the choice of appropriate therapy and care. Each of these decisions can have major resource implications for the health service and consequences for the work of other staff. Yet it is rare for any of them to be directly contradicted or challenged by a manager or by any other occupational group within the NHS. Practical problems (shortage of beds, absence of equipment) can be pointed out, but diagnosis and treatment are finally matters for the doctor. The hospital patient is the patient of a named consultant, not of a manager or a nurse or a medical social worker. This is an expression of what we will term the 'micro-power' of hospital doctors. It is hard to challenge because the key decisions we have referred to are complex and difficult ones, and doctors are the only group trained to the requisite level of expertise. Thus management cannot, for example, simply replace doctors with some other, more compliant group of workers, or with robots or computers.

Both medical micro-power and macro-power are reinforced by cultural factors. The medical profession enjoys high social status and respect – much higher, according to social surveys, than either politicians or managers. There may be some luck in this too – there is a sense in which doctors are lucky to be dealing with conditions in which their clients are dependent on them and frequently *want* to believe in their extreme skill and ethical commitment. This strong 'halo effect' is not enjoyed by, for instance, car salesmen or even schoolteachers. Doctors, both collectively and individually, are able to draw on it as a resource. Occasionally they use it to support their expressions of opinion on what are clearly not *medical* issues at all, such as the allocation of resources between different services.

Nor is it only members of the general public who are culturally predisposed to accept the authority of doctors. Most groups of health service workers are similarly deferential, though the intensity of this deference may well be lessening. Nurses are the best-known case, where much of the development of the profession has been shaped and conditioned by doctors, and where appropriate deference was for long a quite explicit part of the process of nurse socialisation. As mentioned earlier, NHS consultants have managed to create something of a person-culture (Table 1.1) around themselves. The chief surgeon, with his carnation buttonhole, striding through the ward on a 'grand round', pursued by a gaggle of juniors and nurses, is clearly a star.

These cultural factors have helped doctors to achieve their immediate personal aims and preserve their local autonomy with a minimum of overt conflict. They seldom have to insist on their rights or fight for their position because, culturally, the groups with whose interests those of the doctors conflict are defeated on the second and third faces of power before it ever comes to the direct and open competition of the first face.

In so far as nurses believe it is always their job to meet the consultant's wishes (even if this creates difficulties for the nurses or patients) then the potential conflict remains submerged on Lukes' third dimension. In so far as it is used by non-doctors the phrase 'Doctor knows best' is a classic indicator of the presence of third-face medical power.

However, even where nurses, managers and other health workers are conscious of clashes of interest with the medical profession they may rationally choose not to fight. The odds against success or the time and energy needed may make the costs of challenging medical power seem too high. We encountered a number of examples of this among managers during our research into the impact of general management 1983–88 (see Chapter 3). Several managers said that it wasn't worth pushing resource management too hard because of medical resistance. Such exclusion of an issue from formal agendas, or at least relegation of it to a low priority position, is typical of the exercise of second face power.

One major question is whether the new tools which *Working for Patients* has put into the hands of managers will enable them to challenge doctor micropower more effectively than has been the case in the past. If so one might expect issues to move into the first face type of public disagreement and conflict. There have already been some straws in the wind indicating that this may be happening (e.g. O'Sullivan, 1990).

This chapter has attempted to lay out a conceptual and theoretical framework within which the reader is invited to consider the material in later chapters. An explicit reconsideration of the post-Fordist model and its applicability to the future NHS is reserved for the final chapter. In the intervening chapters, however, many of the particular discussions will draw on the contrasting ideas of a Fordist, 'command' approach or a flexible, decentralised strategy more akin to the post-Fordist ideal. In each case it is useful to seek to identify the pre-requisites, in terms of power relationships and the degree of fit of the relevant organisational cultures.

CHAPTER 2

NHS Management Past

PREVIEW

As we noted in the preceding chapter, the central question addressed by this book is why the NHS has been so difficult to reform. Although our final chapter looks at the reforms associated with the white paper, *Working for Patients*, introduced in 1990–91, our particular concern is with the results of that set of reforms, associated with the Griffiths Report of 1983, introduced under the rubric of 'general management' in the mid–1980s. This chapter serves two purposes, to each of which we have devoted one main section of the text.

First, it is necessary to provide a picture of the management of the Service as it was carried on prior to the Griffiths reforms; without this, we cannot, as we attempt in Chapters 3 and 4, assess their impact. The first main section of text therefore draws upon both the history of the formal organisation of the Service, and published empirical research about its management, in order to provide such a benchmark for comparison.

Second, we need to say something about the Griffiths changes themselves. Part of this is a straightforward description of the diagnosis and prescription offered by the Griffiths Report itself, and subsequently extended and implemented by the government. But unless these reforms were in some sense significant, there would be no point in writing this book. In addition, therefore, we assess their potential significance in terms of the key concepts which we introduced in Chapter 1.

This chapter is therefore somewhat long and detailed, though by no means as long or detailed as it could have been; wherever possible we have summarised and provided references to sources of greater detail. What remains is, however, essential for a full understanding of what follows.

NHS MANAGEMENT BEFORE GRIFFITHS

Our account of NHS management prior to the Griffiths changes draws on two main types of sources. In the next subsection we summarise the formal organisational history of the NHS, drawn mostly from official and semi-official documentation or secondary references to it. In the following subsection we turn to an account of NHS managers and their behaviour drawn largely from published academic research.

Organising – and reorganising – the NHS

It is neither necessary nor desirable for our present purposes to give a blow-by-blow account of the development of the formal organisation of the NHS from its creation in 1948 until the appearance, in 1983, of the Griffiths Report; such an account can be found in Harrison (1988, ch. 2). Although there were large-scale reorganisations in 1974 and in 1982, a long series of changes in the arrangements for managing particular professions and services before and between these, and even more numerous reports on topics related to the management and organi-sational formalities of the NHS, the picture which we wish to paint is one of underlying continuity rather than of significant change. Specifically, we draw attention to five elements in this continuity.

First, control over the overall level of finance going into the NHS has remained firmly with the central government throughout the period. Although the mid-1970s saw important changes in the arrangements for distributing financial resources around the country (the 'RAWP' formula and its counterparts in Wales, Scotland and Northern Ireland: Jones and Prowle, 1984, pp. 92–107), and for allowing for the effects of inflation (the introduction of 'cash limits': Hanley *et al.*, 1986, pp. 24–6), the fact that the Service is overwhelmingly financed from general taxation has allowed central government to control annual expenditure. This is both a strength (for obvious reasons) and a weakness, the reasons for which are part of our second element of continuity.

This second element is that, although under its constituent legislation, the (now) Secretary of State had a statutory duty to provide a NHS, he [*sic*] exercises this through statutory bodies acting as his agents in running the Service. Such bodies featured both in the original design and in subse-quent reorganisations. In England (terminology often varies in other parts of the UK) there were originally Regional Hospital Boards, Hospital Man-agement Committees, Boards of Governors (of teaching hospitals), Execu-tive Councils (holding the contracts of GPs and other family practitioners) and Local Health Committees (local authority – community – health ser-vices). These were transformed in 1974 into Regional Health Authorities, Area Health Authorities and Family Practitioner Committees, with Area Health Authorities being replaced by District Health Authorities in 1982. Moreover, despite variations in constitution, the memberships of these bodies have been appointed rather than elected (though sometimes the membership has included local government councillors) to serve on a part-time basis, and have included varying numbers of doctors and nurses (Levitt, 1979, chs 3 and 4; Levitt and Wall, 1984, chs 3 and 4). Full-time, salaried, chief officers have been responsible to these bodies.

This agency relationship (quite different from, at one extreme, that between a Secretary of State and a nationalised industry, and, at the other, that between a Secretary of State and his or her own civil servants) has given rise to what, from a government perspective, are two problems, both recognised early in the history of the NHS. One is that, as was recognised in a dissenting memorandum to the Guillebaud Committee Report of 1956 (Committee of Enquiry, 1956, p. 274) the Secretary of State often lacks line management control over the NHS. Thus, government priorities for health care often have to be written in rather vague or general terms, and have proved difficult to enforce (Haywood and Alaszewski, 1980, ch. 3). The other problem for the government is that, freed from responsibility for raising funds themselves, such bodies and the managers and professionals whom they employ have no disincentive to publicise the perceived inadequacy of resourcing. As Enoch Powell recalled of his period as Minister of Health from 1960–3:

> One of the most striking features of the National Health Service is the continual deafening chorus of complaint which rises day and night from every part of it . . . The universal Exchequer financing of the service endows everyone providing it as well as using it with a vested interest in denigrating it, so that it presents what must be the unique spectacle of an undertaking that is run down by everyone engaged in it. (Powell, 1966)

A third element of continuity is the close relationship, at national level, between the government and the medical profession. This is an example of what has been referred to as *corporatism*.

> Corporatism can be defined as a system of interest representation in which the constituent units are organised into a limited number of singular, compulsory, noncompetitive, hierarchically ordered categories, recognised or licensed (if not created by) the state and granted a deliberate representational monopoly . . . in exchange for observing certain controls on their selection of leaders and articulating of demands and supports. (Schmitter, 1974, p. 96)

Although it does not meet every single element of the above definition, the medical profession, mainly as represented by the British Medical Association (the only officially recognised trade union) and the Royal Colleges and Faculties, is just such a state-licensed élite. The state uses its legislative authority effectively to prohibit non-members of the profession from practising medicine, and the profession undertakes to control and discipline its members in a variety of ways. The BMA and the Royal Colleges (of Physicians, Surgeons, and so on) are in constant and close contact with ministers and officials (Castle, 1980; Crossman, 1977), being consulted on matters going far beyond the narrow terms of employment of their members. (For examples, see Harrison, Hunter and Pollitt, 1990, pp. 109–13; Harrison, 1981, pp. 93–4.)

The relationship between corporatist arrangements of this kind and the power of the medical profession is not straightforward. Whilst it operates, the arrangement gives doctors direct (that is, without going through the medium of managers on health authorities) access to government, with the opportunity both to shape official thinking about policy in general and to veto unwelcome developments. It is therefore a potential vehicle for the exercise of the third and second dimensions of power to which we referred in Chapter 1. But there are two important caveats. One is that a government may, on occasion, choose to circumvent the arrangements as, for instance, when it imposed a new contract on GPs in 1990 (*The Times*, 24 February 1990, p. 1). This suggests that corporatism is as much a cause of medical influence as a source of it, meaning in turn that it could be, or at least could have become, a government *strategy* for relating to the medical profession rather than something forced on the government by the profession. (For a similar analysis of another part of the public service, see Rhodes, 1986). Our other caveat is that none of this necessarily means that the power of the medical profession has been concentrated at national level; our next focus is upon the local, micro, level.

The fourth pre-Griffiths continuity to which we wish to draw attention is that, at local level, formal organisational arrangements have been so designed as to leave doctors (by which, in this context, we mean GPs and hospital consultants) free from day to day management, and to leave members of other clinical professions managed only by other members of their own profession. Thus, despite the fact that the official Farquharson-Lang Report of 1966 (Scottish Health Services Council, 1966) and a report of the (then) Institute of Hospital Administrators (Joint Working Party, 1967) proposed the creation of non-medically qualified chief executive posts, the Service continued to be administered by groups of managers from a mix of professional backgrounds. No one officer was in overall charge, and, as the 1960s and 1970s progressed, more and more occupations developed their own, exclusive, management structures (Harrison, 1988a, 14–17). The apogee of this was the creation, as part of the 1974 reorganisation, of multidisciplinary management teams of chief officers, taking decisions only by consensus, that is, where no member disagreed (DHSS, 1972a, 29–30). Such teams confirmed the professions of nursing and financial management in their *de facto* equality of status with administration. They also provided to their numbers (amongst whose members at the operational level doctors constituted one-half) the formal right of veto. (For a review of consensus teams in the NHS, see Harrison, 1982.)

Despite the involvement of doctors in the team decision-making process, the medical profession itself remained largely outside the subject matter of that process. Organisational arrangements reflected this; GPs remained self-employed in the manner which, albeit with changes of nomenclature, had persisted since 1912, whilst hospital consultants' contracts of employment were, for the most part, held by Regional Health Authorities, rather than by the Districts or Areas in whose institutions they worked.

But at least as important as all these factors has been the doctrine of 'clinical freedom': the notion that a fully-qualified doctor cannot be directed in his or her clinical work. Official commitment to this doctrine, even into the 1980s, can be evidenced by references in official documentation.

Such references indeed predate the creation of the Service; the 1944 Coalition government *White Paper on a National Health Service* stated that 'whatever the organisation, the doctors taking part must remain free to direct their clinical knowledge and personal skill for the benefit of their patients in the way in which they feel to be best' (Ministry of Health, 1944, p. 26). If such a view underpinned the creation of the NHS, it also underpinned its first reorganisation; the preparatory Crossman Green Paper set out a fundamental principle that 'the Service should provide full clinical freedom to the doctors working in it' (DHSS, 1970). The Secretary of State's foreword to the Conservative white paper which set out the firm plans for the 1974 reorganisation of the NHS assured the reader that

> The organisational changes will not affect the professional relationship between individual patients and individual professional workers on which the complex of health services is so largely built. The professional workers will retain their clinical freedom – governed as it is by the bounds of professional knowledge and ethics and by the resources that are available – to do as they think best for their patients. This freedom is cherished by the professions and accepted by the Government. It is a safeguard for patients today and an insurance for future improvements.   (DHSS, 1972b, p. vii)

The subsequent detailed management arrangements went further in linking management to medicine:

> the objective in reorganising the NHS is to enable health care to be improved. Success in achieving this objective depends primarily on the people in the health care professions who prevent, diagnose

and treat disease. Management plays only a subsidiary part, but the way in which the Service is organised and the processes used in directing resources can help or hinder the people who play the primary part. (DHSS, 1972a, p. 9)

Nor had the philosophy for what was to become the 1982 reorganisation changed much; *Patients First* had the following to say

It is doctors, dentists and nurses and their colleagues in the other health professions who provide the care and cure of patients and promote the health of the people. It is the purpose of management to support them in giving that service. (DHSS and Welsh Office, 1979, pp. 1–2)

Such quotations are, of course, selective. The same documents also make references to such matters as the need for efficiency, but what is striking is that they are careful never to imply that *doctors* might need to become more efficient; the inference is rather that it is other, unspecified, groups which need to be controlled in order to maximise resources for medical care. Thus the above quotation from *Patients First* continues: 'The efficient management of the Service is therefore of the highest importance, not least when resources are tight. The more economical it can be, the more resources there will be for patient care'. It is also true that some of the above documents acknowledge that resources are limited and that priorities need to be established. But here again, there is no challenge to medical autonomy; rather, it is assumed that agreed priorities will somehow emerge from discussions. Thus the 1974 management arrangements speak of mechanisms by which doctors can 'contribute more effectively to . . . decision-making' (DHSS, 1972a, p. 10), whilst *Patients First* refers to machinery 'to ensure that the doctor's voice is fully heard' (DHSS and Welsh Office, 1979, p. 17).

There is little evidence to suggest, therefore, that a desire for increased managerial control over doctors, or for more general management control over other clinical professions, was the foundation of changes in NHS management and organisation prior to the Griffiths Report. On the contrary, the views of such figures as Naylor (a Regional Administrator) and Jaques (an academic), both influential in the design of the 1974 organisation structure, were that 'it is not possible to have a . . . "managing director" . . . clinical doctors could not be made subordinate . . . ' (Naylor, 1971, p. 33); . . . 'no such solution is realistically available' (Jaques, 1978, p. 141).

Our fifth and final pre-Griffiths continuity has already been hinted at in some of the preceding pages: an obsession with organisational formalities as the key to 'better management'. More precisely, there was a dominant assumption in the 1960s and 1970s that the improvement of 'inputs' into management, such as career structures, job specialisation, education, and systems (such as planning), was a sufficient condition for improved results. This philosophy was not confined to the NHS (it is, for instance, clearly discernible in the Fulton Report on the Civil Service: Committee on the Civil Service, 1968), but the NHS was the focus of its archetypical manifestation. The 1966 Salmon Report into Nursing took it as axiomatic that the profession's status was too low, and its proposals for a massive hierarchy of nurse managers was its prescription (Ministry of Health and Scottish Home and Health Department, 1966). In the absence of any philosophy of assessing managerial outputs, claims for improved inputs became the strategy by which NHS occupational groups other than medicine sought to advance themselves (Watkin, 1975, p. 349).

These, then, were the pre-Griffiths NHS organisational formalities. In our next subsection we address the question of how far the actual behaviour of NHS managers and professionals coincided with these.

NHS MANAGEMENT PAST: THE MANAGER AS DIPLOMAT

Table 2.1 indicates the scope of over 20 empirical studies conducted prior to the introduction of general management from 1984 onwards. Despite the variety of foci and research methods employed, the findings of those studies are (with a few exceptions, to which we draw attention below) highly consistent and can therefore confidently be regarded as a realistic picture of pre-Griffiths NHS management.

We summarise the findings in terms of four propositions (Harrison, 1988a, p. 31 ff). First, there was a disjunction between ostensible authority and real influence; put crudely, NHS managers were not the most influential actors. Second, managerial agendas were dominated by the need to react to problem situations rather than to pursue objectives. Third, managers were reluctant to question the value of existing patterns of activities and resource allocation, or to propose major changes in them. The corollary of this was that little interest was displayed in the evaluation of services. Fourth, the bulk of managerial attention was devoted to other groups of employees, rather than towards patients, relatives, or the community at large; managers were producer- rather than consumer-oriented.

Managerial Influence before Griffiths

Despite the persistence of the term 'administrator' in pre-Griffiths grades

Table 2.1 Empirical Research in the NHS: 1948–83

AUTHOR(S) AND PUBLICATION DATE	FIELDWORK	SCALE AND SCOPE	METHODS AND SOURCES
FORSYTH (1966)	1954	One RHB & its HMCs	Questionnaire, documents
ROWBOTTOM et al. (1973)	1956–72	One RHB & 9 HMCs	Interviews, action research
COMMITTEE OF ENQUIRY INTO ELY HOSPITAL (1969)	1957–68	One hospital	Formal inquiry
BROWN (1979) BROWN et al (1975) HAYWOOD (1977)	1972–75	One Area Health Authority and its predecessors	Interviews, questionnaires, documents, observation
KLEIN & LEWIS (1976)	1974–75	205 CHCs	Questionnaire
HUNTER (1979, 1980, 1984a)	1975–77	12 Scottish Health Boards	Questionnaire, interviews, documents, observation in 2 Boards
HAM (1981)	1975–77 (re 1948/74)	One RHB	Documents, interviews
HALLAS (1976)	1975–76	17 CHCs, 60 CHC secretaries	Action research
HAYWOOD et al. (1979) HAYWOOD (1979) ELCOCK & HAYWOOD (1980) HAYWOOD & ALASZEWSKI (1980)	1975–78	DHSS, 2 RHAs, 4 AHAs and associated Teams	Documents, interviews, observation

Table 2.1 (Continued)

AUTHOR(S) AND PUBLICATION DATE	FIELDWORK	SCALE AND SCOPE	METHODS AND SOURCES
BARNARD et al. (1979, 1980) LEE & MILLS (1982)	1976–79	2 Area Health Authorities	Documents, interviews, observation
WISEMAN (1979)	1976–78	SHHD, Planning Council, One Scottish Health Board	Documents, interviews, observation
KOGAN et al. (1978)	1977	DHSS, Welsh Office, SHHD, 3 RHAs, 6 Area Authorities, 8 Districts, 6 CHCs (in England, Wales, Scotland & N.Ireland)	Interviews
COMMITTEE OF INQUIRY INTO NORMANSFIELD HOSPITAL (1978)	1978	One hospital	Formal inquiry
HARRISON (1988b) BARNARD & HARRISON (1986)	1978–82	Health Authorities in England	Interviews, questionnaires documents
STEWART et al. (1980)	1979	32 District Administrators 9 Area Administrators	Interviews, observation
HARRISON (1981) HARRISON et al. (1990)	1979–80	DHSS, professional associations	Interviews, documents
HARDY (1986)	1979–80	2 hospital closures	Interviews, documents
STOCKING (1985)	1980–83	22 innovations in general: 4 detailed cases in RHAs and 12 Districts	Interviews, documents questionnaires

Table 2.1 (Continued)

AUTHOR(S) AND PUBLICATION DATE	FIELDWORK	SCALE AND SCOPE	METHODS AND SOURCES
RATHWELL (1987)	1980–83	One HA	Interviews, documents
WEBB et al. (1986) HARDY et al. (1990)	1980–85	2 DHAs, Local Authority	Interviews, documents
GLENNERSTER et al. (1983)	1980–81	2 DHAs, 2 Local Authorities, London	Interviews
SHULZ & HARRISON (1983)	1981	19 Management Teams	Interviews, documents, some observation
HAM (1986)	1981–85	2 DHAs	Action research
HARRISON, HAYWOOD & FUSSELL (1984)	1982	72 managers	Open ended questionnaire
THOMPSON (1986)	1982–84	7 Management Teams	Interviews, documents
HAYWOOD (1983) HAYWOOD & RANADE (1985)	1982–84	6 DHAs (Members)	Documents, interviews, observation, repertory grid
HARRISON, POHLMAN & MERCER (1984) POHLMAN (1985)	1983–84	40 Consultants and 40 GPs in 6 districts	Interviews
FORTE (1986)	1983–84	1 District	Documents, interviews

Source: Adapted from Harrison, (1988a)

and titles in the NHS, the notion that the Service needed better management and that senior administrators and senior members of a number of the health professions should regard themselves as managers pre-dates Griffiths by some 30 years (Harrison, 1988a, ch. 2). Consequently, formal organisational arrangements have typically been expressed in terms of a hierarchy: with authority ostensibly flowing downwards from central government to health authorities, to chief officers, thence to everyone else (see, for example, DHSS 1972a).

The reality, on the contrary, has been that, except in the case of central control over total finance, none of these was the most influential factor. Thus, a number of studies have shown how, despite the existence of central policies and priorities, the strategic shape of the NHS was dominated by the medical profession. Thus, Haywood and Alaszewski (1980, pp. 104–6) examined the pattern of inputs to, and outputs from, the NHS during the 1970s, showing that whilst real resources available (staff, money) rose considerably, output in terms of the number of cases treated (as inpatients or outpatients) rose much more modestly. Although this discrepancy is to some extent due to improvements in staff conditions of employment, the major explanation is increased intensity of diagnosis and treatment, a conclusion confirmed by increases in the workload of pathology, radiology and physiotherapy departments, and by the rising ratio of total attendances to new outpatients. This can be seen as implying a decision, not taken by politicians or managers but by individual clinicians, to devote the majority of additional resources to greater intensity of care rather than to treating larger numbers of patients. That is, the decisions which underlay these aggregates were individual clinicians' decisions about admission, diagnosis, therapy, and discharge. (It should be appreciated, of course, that these conclusions involve no judgement about the value or otherwise of such trends). These observations, together with an analysis of failures to implement national priorities, also led the authors to comment that 'the power of [central government] to effect change is limited, even when only a modest change in emphasis is envisaged' (p. 61), a conclusion supported in Stocking's study of the pattern of introduction of day case surgery (1985, pp. 223–8).

This strategic influence of the medical profession can also be discerned in the arrangements for the education and supply of professional manpower, a crucial resource for the NHS. Harrison's study of this area concluded that the arrangements were to varying degrees dominated by professional organisations rather than by managers or even by the DHSS. Underneath a complex surface pattern of many official and professional bodies was, however, a dominant medical influence; 'the whole mechanism is not nearly as pluralistic as the mere listing of the bodies involved may convey; not only is the medical profession dominant within most of them, but the same sections of the profession . . . are represented within many' (Harrison, 1981, p. 94). Kogan *et al*. (1978, p. 174) have pointed out that decisions by bodies such as the General Medical Council can result in the non-recognition of hospital training posts which in turn can result in hospital closure.

Conclusions about strategic medical influence are also supported by research into the management and policy process in specific NHS Regions. Elcock and Haywood (1980, pp. 77, 97) note that 'in both Regions, the medical profession fought vigorously against changes in priorities intended to favour the [official priority groups of patients] at the expense of the acute sector.' Nor do such conclusions relate solely to the post-reorganisation period. Ham's historical study concluded that legal and financial controls were not an effective means of securing change; 'the capacity of the central [government] department to ensure that its policies were implemented was limited' even though 'its style became more promotional and interventionist as the 1960s progressed' (Ham, 1981, pp. 191–2). Stocking's (1985) study of such longstanding central priorities as Regional Secure Units and the revision of waking times for hospital inpatients confirms this conclusion as does the study of the implementation of mental handicap policy conducted by Hardy *et al*. (1990). Schulz and Harrison's respondents confirmed the perception that the DHSS and RHAs had relatively little influence (1983, pp. 30–3).

The picture remains unchanged when the influence of members of Area and (later) District Health Authorities is examined. Despite the possibility of relatively influential chairpersons, (Haywood and Ranadé, 1985), members were often starved of important information (Brown *et al*., 1975, pp. 11–14), and had little influence on policy, priorities, resource allocation, or specific decisions; their role was largely that of a 'rubber stamp' (Hunter, 1984 p. 50; see also Hunter, 1980, p. 198; Ham, 1986, pp. 123–6; Schulz and Harrison, 1983, p 30; Glennerster *et al*., 1983, p. 261).

If members were not the most influential actors within health authorities, neither were managers. A number of case studies have instanced the influence of hospital consultants on specific decisions. Kogan's research for the Royal Commission on the NHS documented the case of a decision to transfer the responsibility for biomedical engineering to the works officer, twice overturned as a result of medical objections (Kogan *et al*., 1978 p. 129 ff). This ability to veto change was capable of persisting over long periods; Rathwell (1987) has shown how, in one health authority, attempts to settle the number and distribution of hospital beds for the elderly remained unsuccessful, as a result of medical disagreements, over a period of four years. Even a severe winter, and consequent admissions crisis did not aid resolution, which had still not been achieved at the conclusion of the research (*ibid.*, chapter 4). In another study, Linstead has shown how consultant physicians, on this occasion in alliance with another professional group, were able to veto proposed changes in training arrangements for hospital technicians (1984, p. 11). A further example of the obstructive ability of the medical profession is provided in Forte's (1986, p. 43) case study of one district; clinicians were able to delay the implementation of the whole operational plan by withdrawing their earlier agreement to acute service 'rationalisations'. The ability of doctors to impose their definition of a particular situation upon others has been well illustrated by Ham's example of proposed alterations to bed allocations between hospitals being seen as a lack of suitable case material for medical teaching rather than as a need to provide a good service for the elderly (Ham, 1981, pp. 147–9). Glennerster's respondents were reported as well aware of the ability of consultants to cause and prevent change (Glennerster *et al.*, 1983, p. 260)

The overall conclusion to be drawn from these findings is that, in the pre-Griffiths era at least, doctors were the most powerful group in the Service. It is important, however, to note the form taken by this influence. First, it was not (usually) *organised* influence. Certainly it was, in a special sense, collective; individual clinical decisions produced an aggregate 'resultant' (Lindblom, 1979). But this is not an organised, or even conscious, attempt by doctors to exert influence. Second, where conscious attempts were made, they were often defensive; the existing order of influence suited the medical profession (Forsyth, 1966, pp. 128–30; Harrison, Haywood and Fussell, 1984; see also Alford, 1975, p. 14). Third, attempts to sidestep the problem of local medical influence by incorporating and channelling it into management systems have very largely failed, precisely because it is not organised influence. Thus, the elected clinicians on consensus teams did not proxy the influence of their colleagues (Schulz and Harrison, 1983, pp. 26–7), professional advisory machinery was often ineffective because individuals would not surrender their autonomy to it (Brown *et al.*, 1975, pp. 16, 50–1), and professional participation in central government decision making did not guarantee acceptance by the rank and file (Harrison, Hunter and Pollitt, 1990, chapter 4).

The account given above has to a large extent focussed on the relative influence of doctors and managers, which, we argue below, is a crucial issue in examining the impact of the Griffiths reforms. However, it needs also to be noted that, once doctors are disregarded, managers (more precisely, administrators) were the most influential amongst the remaining actors despite the formal equality of nurses. Thus Stewart *et al.* (1980, pp. 35, 81, 83) rated District Administrators as highly influential, partly because of their access to information. Similarly, Schulz and Harrison (1983, p. 24) show that top managers regarded the chief administrator as the most powerful actor, other than hospital consultants, in the resource allocation process. The relative lack of influence of trade unions, at least when confronted by managers competent in political skills, has been shown in Hardy's (1986, p. 11) study of hospital closure and Harrison's (1988b) study of demands for union membership agreements (see also Barnard and Harrison, 1986).

Management as Tackling Problems

The process of management is, of course, closely associated with problem solving; only the most remote and long-term strategic planner could divorce the two, and several studies of top managers in the commercial world have made it clear that their activities are a good deal more fragmented and problem-oriented than the textbook model of the goal-oriented executive might allow (see, for instance, Kotter, 1982; Mintzberg, 1973). The issue, then, is one of degree; *how* proactive were NHS managers, and how far did they seek out impending problems rather than reacting to the ones thrust upon them? It is not reasonable to expect substantial degrees of proactive behaviour at every level of management; one might expect the degree to diminish as the hierarchy is descended. And indeed the evidence from the NHS is that even upper middle managers attending university-based continuing education courses conceived their roles almost exclusively in terms of tackling problems (Harrison, Haywood and Fussell, 1984, p. 146).

The process of planning is where, perhaps, one might most expect to find proactive behaviour; studies of NHS planning show that this was rarely possible. For instance, Barnard *et al.* (1979, Vol. 3, p. 16) document the way in which a London health authority's attempts to assess the health care needs of its population were rapidly abandoned in order to produce 'defensive' information to demonstrate the perceived unfairness to the authority of the RAWP formula. The northern health district studied by Forte (1986, pp. 24–5) experienced similar difficulty in sustaining proactive behaviour. In Scotland, Hunter found ' . . . plans thwarted by the flare-up of a crisis, such as occurred in both [health boards where fieldwork was conducted] over nursing staff establishments' (1980, p. 151), whilst even within the Scottish Home and Health Department planning was reactive and *ad hoc* (Wiseman, 1979, pp. 106–7).

It might also be expected that proactive behaviour would be found in the activities of chief officers of health authorities, and the management teams of which they were members. In their study of District Administrators, Stewart *et al.* (1980, p. 76) note, however, that few were able to play the more proactive roles of shaping plans, innovating new practices or of managing the total organisation; rather the evidence (pp. 149–71) of how the research subjects spent their days shows little sign of interest in strategic issues but a preoccupation with *ad hoc* referrals of issues. Nor was the content of management team agendas any different; Schulz and Harrison (1983, p. 37) note that a major item of team work was 'tackling of issues which in some way presented themselves as problems to the team or its members'. Haywood's systematic classification of the agenda items of several management teams shows the prevalence of non-strategic items (Haywood 1979, pp. 54, 57); 90 per cent of items consisted of information exchange, deciding to whom issues should be referred ('process'), or routine decision-making. Yet the teams were created in order to take 'decisions for the totality of health care' (DHSS 1972a, p. 15). Haywood summarises by describing chief officers as 'directors of process . . . reactors rather than initiators . . . '(1979, p. 59). Hunter's study of decision-making in two Scottish Health Boards reached virtually the same conclusion. The process consisted 'largely of administering and maintaining a system rather than of making fundamental changes in it' (Hunter, 1980, p. 183).

The overall picture, therefore, is one of managerial coping, with little real attention being paid to the implementation of national priorities. In some studies the impression is left that it was tackling (rather than solving) the problem which was important, especially if this involved potential conflict with a doctor (see, for instance, Klein, 1978, p. 1803; Harrison, Haywood and Fussell, 1984, p. 186).

Maintaining the Status Quo

The notion of 'incremental analysis' was coined by Lindblom (1959, 1979) to denote an approach to decision-making which severely limits the extent to which the alternatives considered depart from the existing situation. Such limited analysis was characteristic of pre-Griffiths NHS management.

One way of approaching this is to look at the nature of planning options explored. These show a strong emphasis on hospital beds; thus Rathwell (1987, ch. 4) has shown how planning for the elderly in one authority was largely confined to beds, notwithstanding the existence of official priority for community care. (In the same study, planning for the mentally handicapped, where no beds existed, was not so constrained). Similarly, Ham (1981, p. 147) has shown how in another city the problems of the elderly were perceived as a problem of 'bed blocking' and Glennerster *et al.* (1983, p. 261) have shown the importance with which national norms were treated. Planning options also showed a strong emphasis on what Brown *et al.* termed 'shopping lists of deficiencies' in existing services:

> When the . . . district teams submitted their . . . priorities for long-term development . . . over half concerned the development of primary care . . . [but] when it came to concrete proposals . . . 'community' projects did not fare quite so well . . . They received . . . their pre-reorganisation share of the share-out. (Brown *et al.* 1975, pp. 103–4)

According to Thompson (1986, p. 20), things had not changed by the 1980s. Such *ad hoc* planning was also to be found in Scotland (Wiseman, 1979), though planning documents sometimes sought to conceal this by the inclusion of large quantities of symbolic information unrelated to actual proposals for change (Schulz and Harrison, 1983, p. 38). Glennerster *et al.* (1983, p. 264) note that most of the respondents in their study 'still thought of planning as what to do with the increment' and also provide an insight into why this should be so; 'in theory, people favoured a change in priorities but only on the basis of "you can do it so long as you don't touch me"' (p. 260). A further characteristic of planning options follows closely from this. Hunter (1980, pp. 145, 184) notes that development funds were not merely regarded as important, but for many actors were the answer to planning problems; the tendency was always to seek more resources rather than to question the value of existing resource use; most developments were the result of building schemes, and most also meant 'more of the same'.

An alternative way of looking at the matter is to note the general absence of review or evaluation from even senior management activity (Brown, 1979, p. 205; Lee and Mills, 1982, p. 179). The management teams in Schulz and Harrison's study allocated resources incrementally; when asked individually about their objectives, respondents overwhelmingly replied that they were concerned, first, to keep existing services intact, and, second, to respond if possible to internal demands for expansion. Movement towards national priorities came only in third place (Schulz and Harrison, 1983, p. 37). Not surprisingly, therefore, Barnard *et al.* (1979, Vol. 3, p. 32) found that 'little attention was paid to collecting information on resource use . . . or on outcomes'. To some extent, however, the illusion of scrutiny was maintained by such devices as frequent visits to institutions by senior officers, though these were in practice quite uncritical in approach (Schulz and Harrison, 1983, p. 37); there is clearly no necessary connection between critical evaluation and the practice of 'management by wandering about' (Peters and Waterman, 1982, p. 121ff). In a more recent study Thompson (1986, p. 57) was surprised to observe 'the noticeable absence of any systematic monitoring . . . of policy formulation and implementation'.

A final point to note is that this limitation in analytical scope for the most part enabled managers to avoid conflict with the medical profession. That there is an apparent contradiction between the logics of professional autonomy and managerial control does not necessarily entail empirical conflict; the evidence does not support the assertions of authors such as Heller (1979, pp. 1, 45) and Petchey (1986, p. 100) that such conflict has been a major force in shaping the NHS. Rather, the suggestion is that when medico-managerial conflict did occur it was often the result of managers being faced with conflicting demands from the profession (Green, 1975, p. 133).

Producer Orientation

We noted above that pre-Griffiths NHS managers were largely problem-oriented in their work. A natural question to ask would therefore be, what kinds of problem and what other actors? The notion of introversion summarises the answer to this question; both the sources and nature of management problems were to be found inside the organisation, rather than outside it in the form of patients, relatives or public. In other words managerial action was producer-led rather than consumer-led.

First, it can be established that Community Health Councils (CHCs), the official representatives of the health care consumer, had relatively little impact. Hallas concluded from his research in one Region that:

> On the whole, Councils have been far too polite and deferential . . . the tendency [is] to accept information on trust . . . to assume that if persons have a string of qualifications and/or resounding titles, then they are not to be deferred to, even in matters which are not within their professional competence.   (Hallas, 1976, p. 59)

And CHCs were reluctant to use the modest formal authority that they had been given in 1974:

> With rare exceptions they accepted, without much demur, proposals for closing down hospitals and wards: a pattern which is all the more interesting since this is one of the few areas of activity where CHCs actually have some power, even if it is only the power of delay.   (Klein and Lewis, 1976, p. 135)

These studies occurred in the early days of CHCs, and it is certainly the case that they subsequently became much more active in resisting closures (Allsop, 1984, p. 197). However, by the 1980s CHCs were still reporting difficulty over getting acceptance for their notion of 'consultation' (Ham, 1980, p. 226), and top managers regarded them as uninfluential (Schulz and Harrison, 1983, p. 30–3). Writing of the consultation process of which CHCs were only a part, Lee and Mills concluded

(1982, p. 142) that 'few of those [bodies] consulted perceived much benefit to be gained from the formal consultation process'.

Second, studies of NHS managers' behaviour show that their attention was strongly focussed within the organisation rather than outwards. Stewart *et al.* (1980, pp. 172–7) traced all issues with which District Administrators dealt over a three-day period, almost none of which did not originate within the health authority. Similarly, all the examples of decisions quoted in Haywood's study (1979, pp. 57–8) are internal in origin. The Howe Report into the scandal at Ely hospital had shown a closed community with no awareness of standards elsewhere and an inbuilt resistance to complaints (Committee of Enquiry, 1969, p. 115 ff) (and this was not the first or last such scandal), so that Thompson's comment from a study conducted in the early 1980s is apposite:

> One of the more sobering features of the study was an apparent lack of interest in consumer responses, even the relevance and significance of patients' complaints.   (Thompson, 1986, p. 57)

The same kind of inward orientation was evident in the work of upper middle managers; administrators and nurse managers largely defined their work agendas in terms of, respectively, tackling problems raised by other groups of workers, and devising improved organisational formalities (Harrison, Haywood and Fussell, 1984, p. 1987).

Summary: Power and Culture in the Pre-Griffiths NHS

There is a considerable degree of consonance between the formal organisational characteristics of the NHS, as we outlined them in the first part of this chapter, and the behaviour of NHS managers and professionals as revealed in the research studies which we have cited. (We do not argue, incidentally, that one 'causes' the other; the reality is far more complex, and iterative). Moreover, the picture of the pre-Griffiths NHS manager which emerges from the research is a fairly coherent one in which the prime tasks are problem-solving, organisation maintenance, and the facilitation of processes. It has been given the label 'diplomat' (Harrison, 1988a, p. 51). Although the research provides evidence of occasional exceptions to this role (which we shall discuss in a moment), the respective cultures of NHS management and medicine had a good deal of common content (Schulz and Harrison, 1983 p. 44; Brown, 1979, p. 79, 191), resting *inter alia* on acceptance of the notion of 'clinical freedom', that is, that third party (including government and managers') restrictions on the doctor-patient relationship should be minimal, or at most confined to control over aggregate resources (Harrison, 1988a, p. 5; Harrison, Pohlman and Mercer, 1984). This common culture had, it may be noted, elements of both the Fordist model (for instance, in its emphasis on procedural conformity and assumption of permanent, career employment) and the post-Fordist model (in respect of the autonomy accorded to local groups and networks and the resistance to standardisation of the production process). (See Table 1.2).

These shared aspects of culture were closely linked to the predominant form of medical power. Although, as we have seen, some overt conflict occurred, manifest in obstructive behaviour by hospital consultants (an example of what we referred to in Chapter 1 as the 'first dimension' of power), our interpretation is that it is the 'second dimension' which was more pervasive; doctors were able to keep the threat of major changes to the status quo off the agenda. Perhaps also, as Haywood and Alaszewski (1980, p. 137) have argued, the 'third dimension' is discernible in 'clinical freedom': in effect the power to define what is possible. Indeed, it is our view that, of the four propositions employed above to summarise the research findings, it is the first (the one about medical power) that is, as it were, an independent variable. In other words, the fact that managers were relatively uninfluential in relation to doctors meant that the former were unable to be strategists, unwilling to question the status quo, and unable to give priority to anything other than problems raised from within the organisation. What, then, are the prospects of a successful challenge to such power? Any attempt to shift NHS management away from the diplomat role would represent a challenge to medical power, and its success would be crucially dependent upon the effectiveness of such a challenge. There are two, complementary approaches to such a question.

The first approach is concerned with the motivations of the relevant actors: first, the managers. Although, as we have shown, there was a very great deal of homogeneity in the findings of empirical studies of pre-Griffiths NHS management, we should note that a number of them did produce some exceptions: examples of management behaviour which was less reactive and less incremental than the norm. This tiny minority of counter examples has, unfortunately, not been well analysed by the authors of the studies in which they occur. Thus Stewart *et al.* (1980, p. 78 ff) do not explain why a few of their District Administrators were able to be proactive. Nor do Schulz and Harrison (1983, pp. 40–3) offer much explanation for why a few of their management teams were able to be proactive, beyond suggesting a degree of pragmatism and some kind of synergy involving a respected medical officer. Rathwell's case study of mental handicap is a little better in this respect; he argues that the successful relationship between a joint care planning team, a local authority and voluntary organisations was made possible by its situation within a health authority where there were no existing mental handicap beds, and therefore no medical vested interests at stake (Rathwell, 1987, chs 4, 8). Also, Hunter in his study of decision-making and the allocation of development funds notes that the scope for innovation and change was not wholly absent. He cites the emphasis given to community health services as an example of how pressures for policy change can combine to bring about breaks in precedent (Hunter, 1980, p. 174). It is not, of course, now possible for us to explain these exceptions. But we refer to them in order to show that no 'iron law of diplomacy' shaped pre-1983 NHS management. Indeed, there were two factors which might be seen to have offered the possibility of change. First, despite the shared culture to which we have referred, many managers were also frustrated with their role (Stewart et al., 1979, pp. 30, 66, 113, 117–18; Haywood et al., 1979, pp. 26, 35, 39; Schulz and Harrison, 1983, p. 17; Fairey et al., 1975, pp. 25–6; Klein, 1984, p. 1708).

Second, there was the issue of doctors' motivation: there is evidence that the view of clinical freedom held by the medical profession might have been somewhat more elastic than is sometimes suggested. From their study of doctors' conceptions of the notion, Harrison et al. conclude

[C]linical freedom seems to be primarily of symbolic or polemical importance; it is not conceived of as absolute and existing 'breaches' are for the most part quickly accepted and rationalised. The notion is seen as more relevant to prospective 'breaches' . . . [I]t implies that managerial innovations will be able to make significant inroads into clinical freedom provided that the pace of change is not too rapid to prevent acceptance and rationalisation.   (Harrison, Pohlman and Mercer, 1984, p. 11, emphasis added)

In general, therefore, managers *might* be willing to challenge, and doctors *might* be willing to concede.

But we need also to examine the matter from a more fundamental perspective; what is the basis of professional power, especially medical power? It will be recalled from Chapter 1 that we identified dependence as the logical corollary of power; when we ask about the basis of professional power in relation to NHS managers, we therefore ask about the ways in which the latter are dependent upon the former. A number of answers can be given. An obvious one is that professionals have expert knowledge and skills upon which members of the public are dependent and which NHS managers cannot themselves supply directly. Another answer is that professionals bestow legitimacy upon the NHS as a whole, including its managers; this is partly a matter of luck (helping the sick is seen as a worthwhile activity), though doctors and nurses, particularly, have been able to combine this with their ability to alleviate distress, so as to develop an authoritative position in public opinion. (For a selection of opinion polls concerning this, see Harrison, 1988a, pp. 88–9.)

Perhaps more fundamentally than this, and recalling our discussion of puzzlement and uncertainty in Chapter 1, the medical profession seems to have a special power base, which arises from the ability of doctors to deal with what would otherwise be major uncertainties for managers (cf. Hinings *et al.*, 1971); they have the ability to ration health care. Briefly, the reasoning behind our analysis is as follows; for an elaboration, see Harrison, (1988a, ch. 1).

First, it is axiomatic that resources are finite; resources for health care cannot therefore be infinite. Second, under conditions (such as in the NHS) where users do not pay directly for health care, demand is potentially infinite. (Even if this is not so, experience in other countries suggests that demand can be several times greater than the level currently being met in the UK). In practice, demand is fuelled by, amongst other things, developments in medical technology and the dependence of an increasingly aged population (for more details see Harrison, 1988a, ch. 5). Third, and as a result of the preceding two factors, rationing of health care necessarily occurs and will continue to do so; there will be people who want (and would benefit from) health care, but to whom it will be denied. The important questions concern the *criteria* used to ration care (a matter which we cannot discuss here; see, for instance, Boyd, 1979), and the *process* by which it is achieved.

Fourth, one important process for NHS rationing is explicit queueing: waiting lists. But this is clearly not an option for urgent medical needs, and, even in respect of less urgent needs has become a major source of public criticism of the government, and the NHS managers, in the 1980s. Fairly clearly, no one has much to gain by being seen to deny care; one way of avoiding being thus seen is to leave it to doctors, who not only have the benefit of public legitimacy, but can, under the rubric of clinical freedom, make rationing decisions largely invisible. As two US researchers of the NHS illustrated it:

> By various means, physicians . . . try to make the denial of care seem routine or optimal. Confronted by a person older than the prevailing unofficial age of cut-off for dialysis, the British GP tells the victim of chronic renal failure or his family that nothing can be done except to make the patient as comfortable as possible in the time remaining. The British nephrologist tells the family of a patient who is difficult to handle that dialysis would be painful and burdensome and that the patient would be more comfortable without it.   (Aaron and Schwartz, 1984, p. 101)

This, of course, is no more than a specific, albeit dramatic, example of the research findings to which we referred in the preceding section; the pattern of health services provided by the NHS is largely the aggregate of individual clinical decisions. Doctors, left to themselves, can solve problems which managers (and politicians) have found difficult. As our analysis proceeds through Chapters 5 and 6 we shall return to this matter of managerial dependence upon professionals. Now, however, we turn to the Griffiths changes in general.

GRIFFITHS AND ITS SIGNIFICANCE

We begin our analysis of the Griffiths changes with a brief account of the circumstances leading up to the report, its diagnosis and prescription, and the steps taken by the government as a result. (For a fuller account, including an explanation of the pressures that led to these events, see Harrison, 1988a, chs 5, 6). We also need to show, however, that the Griffiths changes are potentially important enough to warrant our writing this book. The final section of this chapter is therefore devoted to an analysis of the differences between the Griffiths and related proposals and the culture and behaviour which preceded them.

Griffiths: Diagnosis and Prescription

We begin our account with a number of managerial developments which, though they pre-date the Griffiths Report, very much reflect its potential challenge to the old culture.

From 1981 onwards the NHS had been expected by the government to make 'efficiency savings'; this practice consisted of assuming that health authorities' outturn expenditure would be less than their nominal budget by a specified percentage, and hence providing an actual budget to match only the assumed outturn, but the announcements made by the then new Secretary of State, Mr Norman Fowler, in January 1982 of arrangements to 'improve accountability' in the NHS represented something altogether more sophisticated. There were two elements to these arrangements: a review process and a set of performance indicators.

The review process was intended to secure greater adherence to national policies and priorities than had previously been the case;

> each year Ministers will lead a Departmental review of the long-term plans, objectives and effectiveness of each Region with the Chairmen of the Regional Authorities and other Chief Regional Officers. The aims of the new system will be to ensure that each Region is using the resources allocated to it in accordance with the Government's policies – for example giving priority to services for the

elderly, the handicapped and the mentally ill – and also to establish agreement . . . on the progress and development which the Regions will aim to achieve in the ensuing year.   (DHSS, 1982)

A similar process was to take place between Regional Health Authorities and DHAs within each Region. The new process commenced immediately.

Performance indicators were to be developed and employed in conjunction with the review process; they would

enable comparison to be made between districts and so help Ministers and the Regional Chairmen . . . to assess the performance of their constituent . . . authorities in using manpower and other resources efficiently.   (DHSS, 1982)

Unlike earlier attempts to use comparative data, the new indicators were therefore to be compulsory. The first national (English) package of indicators was made available in September 1983, in a form which allowed any health authority to be compared with all others in terms both of absolute values of the indicators used and of rankings within the region and the country. The package contained some 70 indicators relating to clinical work, finance, manpower [sic], support services and estate management, all constructed from already available data. The clinical indicators related mainly to the use of clinical facilities within broad specialty groups, rather than to the outcomes of treatment, consisting of such efficiency measures as average length of hospital stay, throughput of patients per bed per annum, turnover interval between cases occupying a bed, and the ratio of return outpatient visits to new outpatients. They were, however, all measures which are largely determined by the aggregate of doctors' behaviour rather than by managers' decisions.

Less than two months after the original review process/performance indicator announcement, Mr Fowler announced two further initiatives. First, a national enquiry was established with the aim of 'identify[ing] underused and surplus land and property, and, where appropriate dispos[ing] of it'. The subsequent Ceri Davies Report recommended a system of notional rents for NHS property as the basis of a performance measure of estate utilisation and the disposal of unused and underused assets; it was accepted by the Government in November 1983. The other initiative was the experimental use of private firms of accountants to audit the accounts of health authorities.

Only three weeks after this announcement, came the announcement of yet another initiative: the extension of 'Rayner Scrutinies' from the civil service to the NHS. Named after Sir Derek Rayner, Managing Director of Marks and Spencer and part-time efficiency adviser to the

Government, such scrutinies involved intensive study of a particular area of expenditure by an officer seconded from normal duties. Further initiatives followed. In August a Review of NHS Audit arrangements was announced; the results, promulgated a year later, emphasised the need for greater attention to be given to 'value for money' rather than to narrow financial propriety. On 6 October 1982, Mr Fowler informed the Conservative Party Conference that:

> we want manpower [sic] directed at serving the patient, not at building new empires of paper and bureaucracy . . . with this in mind I intend to establish a small team, headed by people from private industry, to achieve it. Their jobs will not be to produce a lengthy report . . . but to help us produce results, not in years but in months.   (Fowler, 1982)

The following day saw the announcement that a firm of chartered accountants was to study the possibility of cash-limiting FPC budgets.

In January 1983, central control of NHS manpower numbers was announced and in February came the first public suggestion that the Government was seriously considering restrictions on doctors' rights to prescribe; in November 1984 the withdrawal occurred from NHS prescription of a range of proprietary drugs which had been previously freely available. On 8 September 1983, health authorities were instructed to engage in competitive tendering for laundry, domestic, and catering services, and in December the Minister for Health announced proposals to place restrictions on the use of deputising services by off-duty GPs.

On 3 February 1983, towards the conclusion of the spate of initiatives outlined above, a development occurred which was to crystallise and symbolise the post-1982 policy for managing the NHS. The Secretary of State announced that:

> Four leading businessmen are to conduct an independent management Inquiry into the effective use and management of manpower and related resources in the National Health Service . . . we are setting the Inquiry two main tasks: to examine the way in which resources are used and controlled inside the health service, so as to secure the best value for money and the best possible services for the patient [and] to identify what further management issues need pursuing for these important purposes . . . Mr Griffiths has not been asked to prepare a report . . . we could simply have set up another Royal Commission and then sat back for several years to await its lengthy report, but on past experience that would not lead to effective action. Instead, we have gone straight for management action, with the minimum of fuss or formality.   (DHSS, 1983)

Mr Roy Griffiths was Deputy Chairman and Managing Director of J Sainsbury, and his inquiry's terms of reference were substantially wider than those announced to the Conservative Party in the previous autumn (see above: for an explanation of the agenda shift, see Harrison, 1988a, pp. 100–4). The Inquiry Team, who conducted their investigation by field visits and discussions rather than by formal hearings, led to a final report, in the form of a 24 page letter (NHS Management Inquiry 1983), to the Secretary of State on 6 October 1983, the full text being made public on 25 October. Despite the Team's lack of interest in academic research findings, their diagnosis of management in the NHS bore an astonishing resemblance to the research-based picture of the pre-Griffiths NHS which we outlined above. There were four elements.

First, the Team were concerned that individual management accountability could not be identified. Management by formal and informal consensus led to 'lowest common denominator decisions' and long delays in the management process: it was difficult to know who was in charge. Second, the 'machinery of implementation [was] generally weak', management lacked thrust and change was very difficult to secure. Third, there was a lack of performance orientation in the Service: little objective-setting and almost no evaluation of services. Fourth, managers lacked concern for consumers' views of the Service. The correspondence between this analysis and the research findings to which we referred above is set out in Table 2.2.

The Team's prescription was baldly stated in eight pages. First, changes within DHSS were proposed: the creation of a Health Services Supervisory Board (chaired by the Secretary of State, and including the Minister for Health, the Permanent Secretary, the Chief Medical Officer, the Chairman [sic] of the NHS Management Board (see below), and two or three non-executive members with general management skills and experience) with strategic responsibility for the objectives and resources of the NHS, and, responsible to it, a full-time, multi-professional NHS Management Board to oversee implementation of the strategy. Hence the Management Board would assume all pre-existing NHS management responsibilities located in the DHSS, and its members would include some from outside the civil and health services. Incentives and sanctions in management were held to require attention, and accordingly great stress was placed on the role of a personnel director as a Board member.

Second, general managers were proposed for RHA, DHA and Unit levels of organisation; regardless of discipline, such persons were to carry overall management responsibility for achieving the relevant health authority's objectives, and were to have substantial freedom to design local organisational structures. Functionally-based management structures were to be minimised and day-to-day decisions taken at unit level

Table 2.2   The correspondence between academic research findings and the Griffiths diagnosis

ACADEMIC RESEARCH	GRIFFITHS 'DIAGNOSIS'
Management influence low in relation to clinical professions and medicine in particular	. . . it appears to us that consensus management can lead to *lowest common denominator decisions* and to long delays in the management process . . . In short, if Florence Nightingale were carrying her lamp through the corridors of the NHS today, she would almost certainly be searching for the people in charge (NHS Management Inquiry 1983, pp. 17, 22).
Managerial emphasis is on reacting to problems	. . . . there is no driving force seeking and accepting direct and personal responsibility for developing management plans, securing their implementation and monitoring actual achievement . . . certain major initiatives are difficult to implement . . . [and] above all . . . lack of a general management process means that it is extremely difficult to achieve change . . . [A] more thrusting and committed style of management . . . is implicit in all our recommendations (pp. 12, 19).
Maintenance of the status quo	[The NHS] lacks any real continuous evaluation of its performance . . . rarely are precise management objectives set; there is little measurement of health output; clinical evaluation of particular practices is by no means common and economic evaluation of these practices is extremely rare (p.10).
Producer orientation	Nor can the NHS display a ready assessment of the effectiveness with which it is meeting the needs and expectations of he people it serves. . . . Whether the NHS is meeting the needs of the patient, and the community, and can prove that it is doing so, is open to question (p 10)

Source   Adapted from Harrison (1988a)

rather than higher up the organisation. Thirdly, the review process (see above) was to be extended to unit level, and efficiency savings (see above) replaced by 'cost-improvement programmes', aimed at reducing costs without impairing services.

Fourth, clinical doctors were to become more involved in local management. The prime vehicle for this was a proposed system of 'management budgets': the allocation of workload-related budgets to consultants. The locus of consultant contracts was, however, to remain unchanged. Finally, the Report urged that more attention be paid to patients' and community opinion, expressed through both Community Health Councils and market research methods. The Report also spoke approvingly of some of the earlier initiatives such as performance indicators, the disposal of surplus property, Rayner Scrutinies, and annual reviews.

On the same day as the release of the Report, the Secretary of State for Social Services told the House of Commons that the Government welcomed the thrust of the recommendations and accepted those applicable within the DHSS; the remainder were to be the subject of a short period of consultation. In the event, this period included an investigation by the House of Commons Social Services Committee, whose conclusions were by no means wholly supportive. In general, the comments of medical, nursing and ancillary staff representative organisations were unfavourable whilst those of administrators' and treasurers' organisations were favourable. Unsurprisingly, most comment was directed at the proposal to appoint general managers (Social Services Committee, 1984).

In June 1984, the Secretary of State promulgated the Government's decisions on the Griffiths Report. Some changes, including those within the DHSS and pilot schemes for management budgets, were confirmed as in progress already and the principle of individual general managers in place of consensus teams was accepted: general managers were to be appointed at Regional, District and Unit levels of organisation by the end of 1985; the posts were to be open to NHS managers of all disciplines, to doctors, and to persons from outside the Service. Appointments were to be on the basis of fixed-term contracts of three to five years with renewal for further fixed terms by mutual agreement and, by implication, dependent upon an assessment of the incumbent's performance. Any costs incurred by appointments were to be offset by savings on other management costs.

The Health Services Supervisory Board and the NHS Management Board took a slightly different form from that envisaged in the Griffiths Report. Pressure from the nursing profession led to the early addition of the DHSS Chief Nursing Officer to the Supervisory Board, and only one non-executive outsider, Mr Griffiths himself, was appointed. Mr Victor Paige, formerly Chairman of the Port of London Authority was appointed as Chairman of the NHS Management Board in December 1984 but resigned in June 1986 in circumstances which suggested that there had been difficulties in reconciling political and managerial considerations on such issues as efficiency savings. A revised arrangement resulted, with the Minister for Health as Chairman of the Management Board, (by then Sir) Roy Griffiths as Deputy Chairman (with direct access to the Prime Minister), and Mr Len Peach (Personnel Director of Messrs IBM [UK] as Chief Executive. The composition of the Management Board varied between 1984 and 1987, with roughly one-third of its members from a commercial background, one quarter from the NHS, and the remainder from the civil service.

General managers were appointed by RHAs and DHAs and at Units, though not without suggestions of political 'interference' in ensuring that a number of persons from outside the NHS obtained posts (Timmins, 1985). Nevertheless, more than 60 per cent of posts initially went to former administrators and treasurers. Many of the doctors appointed were clinicians who undertook a part-time management role at unit level, whilst a significant number of appointments from outside the NHS were retiring officers of the armed forces. Subsequent general manager appointments were on rolling, rather than fixed-term contracts, and a system of individual performance review and performance-related pay was introduced. The review process, described earlier, was extended to all levels of the Service, and modified to consist at regional level of a management meeting between the NHS Management Board and officers of each RHA for the review of progress on plans and cost-improvement programmes: this to be followed by a ministerial meeting with chair-persons of individual RHAs with discussion of more strategic and long-term issues, along with major issues arising from the management meeting (Mills, 1987).

By 1992 management budgets still had not been introduced on a widespread basis. Four health districts were chosen as 'demonstration sites' even before the publication of the Griffiths Report, but despite the involvement of management consultants not all of these were successful at the technical level of establishing the necessary information systems. Moreover, they did not gain the widespread support of clinicians. A second generation of demonstrations began in 1985; it was intended that this would pay more attention to the behavioural aspects of such systems. Nevertheless, there remained problems in convincing doctors of the value of the innovation and a further set of pilots proved to be necessary; these were launched in November 1986 under the new name of 'resource management' (Pollitt et al., 1988). Although an evaluation study had been commissioned by the Department of Health, a major extension of resource management was decided upon by the Government as part of the Working for Patients changes (see Chapter 6) long before the (somewhat ambivalent) results of the study were available (Buxton et al., 1989; 1991).

A Management Revolution?

It is often taken for granted that the Griffiths changes to NHS man-agement represented a revolutionary departure from past practice. The grounds on which this assertion is made are often unstated; the case, how-ever, needs to be made explicitly, for as we have shown, organisational and management arrangements have been a matter of fairly constant discussion, and a good deal of change, almost since the inception of the NHS. Strong and Robinson have expressed the intent behind the Griffiths changes in terms of a vision:

> this was not just another way of structuring the health service, it was also a crusade . . . general management . . . was an efficiency drive . . . but . . . it was also, or so it was hoped, a far better way of running health services; a way in which higher quality care would be delivered from co-ordinated frontline workers. Down the tatty corridors of the NHS, new and dedicated heroes would stride – the general managers. Inspired by their leadership a new sort of staff would arise. Armed with better information and new techniques from the private sector, much more closely monitored yet working as a team, they would at last take collective pride in their work – and responsibility for it.   (Strong and Robinson, 1990, p. 3)

It is undoubtedly the case that the Griffiths reforms were implemented with more 'hype' and greater government commitment – and less tolerance of potential dissenters (Pollitt, Harrison, Hunter and Marnoch, 1990, p. 180) – than were earlier reorganisations, and the above quotation certainly encapsulates the way in which managers 'sold' Griffiths to themselves and others. We argue, more specifically, that there are two crucial potential breaks with past practice.

First, a number of the post–1982 changes represent a very clear change to the philosophy of 'diplomatic' management. The most obvious example is the creation of general manager posts and the concomitant loss of professional influence generally, and specifically of the medical veto on the former management teams. That doctors themselves saw the new developments in this light is evident from the BMA's statement to the Social Services Committee:

> it would be very unwise to introduce a single solution on April 1st on what I think are the lines of the Griffiths Report, particularly if it is in conflict with the advice of several professions. It would appear that is the case . . . My assessment of my profession . . . is they would not be prepared to accept an instruction from a lay administrator if they thought it was going to damage the interests of their patients. We are a team of caring professionals, working together, working our way through problems, reaching a consensus and then feeling in honour bound to implement those solutions. If an alternative was imposed upon us, that an executive carried out a policy which was, in our view, damaging to the patient's care, then that choice would not work, sir.   (Social Services Committee, 1984, pp. 4–7)

Nor were the proposals well received by the nursing profession: the Royal College of Nursing launched a national advertising campaign against the notion that general managers would be in charge of nursing (Owens and Glennerster, 1990, p. 4). Many other initiatives from the mid-1980s also challenge the previous philosophy. The review process was intended to procure a shift in *de facto* priorities, away from those of the most prestigious sections of the medical profession (the acute specialties) and towards less prestigious areas such as the elderly, mentally ill and mentally handicapped. Clinical performance indicators reflect the way in which hospital consultants manage their beds and their workload and therefore allows this limited aspect of their performance to be visible to others. Direct management access to consumer and community opinion (through market surveys, for instance) represents a challenge to the widespread assumption that only doctors may legitimately speak on behalf of patients or be aware of their needs. Systems of management budgets/resource management can, if measures of casemix severity are introduced, be used as a vehicle for imposing management priorities on clinicians and for controlling the costs of each type of case.

This changed approach to managing the NHS has been nicely expressed by Day and Klein as a

> move from a system that is based on the mobilisation of consent to one based on the management of conflict – from one that has conceded the right of groups to veto change to one that gives the managers the right to override objections.   (Day and Klein, 1983, p. 1813)

The above measures may provide the potential for managerial influence over doctors, but no such influence will be exerted without appropriate managerial motivation. This is the second element which we identify in the Griffiths revolution: a shift from the philosophy that 'better management' would result from improving the lot of NHS managers (by such means as the provision of appropriate career structures and education), to one which implies that personalised incentives and sanctions are the appropriate motivators. Whilst the pre-Griffiths NHS virtually guaranteed that the clinical professions other than medicine would develop in terms of both occupational role and status, and self-management, the Griffiths changes formally subordinate them to the decisions of general managers. Moreover, the emphasis now is on incentives and sanctions related to managerially and organisationally-defined performance. The whole paraphernalia of performance indicators, short-term contracts, individual performance review and performance-related pay represents a revolutionary departure.

General management can therefore be seen as, in principle, the antithesis of the 1974 system of consensus team decision-making; just as this was a device for both maintaining professional autonomy of doctors and for maintaining the career aspirations of the other clinical professions, so the advent of general management threatened both. In terms of the models that we presented towards the end of Chapter 1, the Griffiths changes represent something of a swing from a mixed mode to one that is more clearly 'Fordist' in character. In Chapters 3 and 4 we examine how far such a shift has actually occurred.

CHAPTER 3

General Management in the NHS: Assessing the Impact

In this chapter we describe, and present the results of, a major study into post-Griffiths management which we conducted between 1987 and 1989 (mainly in 1988).

AIMS AND DESIGN OF THE RESEARCH

In undertaking the research our principal aims were:

- to describe the work that general managers were doing, since research into their behaviour was surprisingly limited (Hunter, 1985)
- to map the perceptions of senior NHS managers – and other senior staff – concerning the impact, or impacts, of general management
- to ascertain whether there were systematic differences in the impact of general management as between one health authority and another, and to explain any such differences
- to review and develop theories of organisation within the NHS.

We adopted a research design that was primarily, but not exclusively, ethnographic (for fuller details see Pollitt *et al.*, 1990). Our ability to conduct a 'before-and-after' study was limited by the variety of reliable descriptions of what had happened 'before'. An experimental approach was ruled out by our inability to control the relevant variables, and by the absence of any control group (since general management had been introduced everywhere there were no health authorities that had not received the 'treatment'). Finally, the objectives of the reform (described in Chapter 2) had in any case only been specified in a loose, quantitative manner. For all these reasons an ethnographic approach seemed most appropriate.

The research was conducted in 11 health authorities (9 English DHAs in 3 RHAs and 2 Scottish Health Boards). We decided to pitch most of our investigations at district and unit levels, but also to strengthen our contextual understanding by conducting selected interviews at regional levels and with senior officials and ministers in central government who were, or had been, connected with the Department of Health and Social Security (DHSS, from 1988 the Department of Health) and the Scottish Home and Health Department (SHHD). A total of 339 interviews (plus numerous informal conversations) were conducted between September 1986 and October 1989 – 98% of these before the end of 1988. Of this total, 301 were at or below district level (or board level in Scotland), 11 were at regional level, and 21 were with officials or politicians of the central departments. The remaining 6 interviews were with officers of a variety of national bodies such as the Royal College of Nursing and the Scottish Hospital Advisory Service.

We selected the districts in which the interviews were to take place according to a variety of criteria. We chose a mixture of large and small, urban and rural, northern and southern and, perhaps most importantly, 'well-resourced' and 'under-funded'. This last dimension we determined by the crude but convenient expedient of examining where districts were in relation to their Resource Allocation Working Party (RAWP) targets. (The RAWP formula, and its Scottish counterpart, were in force throughout the period of our fieldwork.) A health authority which was 'above target' had, in the view of the centre, more resources than it needed. Conversely, a 'below target' authority would be a candidate for assistance when the annual redistribution exercise took place. When we began the research we at least half-expected to find general management having a 'rougher ride' in below-target than above-target authorities though, as will subsequently be explained, this correlation was not supported by our eventual findings. Our selection was therefore determined by the application of these criteria, constrained by our available time and money and guided, to a limited extent, by a preference for authorities where, through previous contacts, we already had 'a foot in the door'.

METHODS

In each of the eight districts and two boards we carried out an average of 37 long, loosely-structured interviews, averaging more than an hour in duration. Our aim was to interview the general manager, other officers on the District Management Board (DMB) or equivalent, a selection of consultants, nurses, the health authority chair and two or more members, Community Health Council representatives, local trade union officials and local authority social services staff. We guaranteed that the identities of the health authorities would remain confidential. In most of the interviews we began with broad, open-ended questions designed to bring out interviewees' own conceptualisations of the Griffiths changes. Later, if necessary, we raised specific issues: for example, what did they think of the Individual Performance Review system (IPR)? We supplemented the interviews with attendance at, and observation of, a number of meetings, and with extensive study of documents, both published plans and internal memoranda. For example, in several of our fieldwork authorities we collected the job descriptions and statements of IPR objectives for key managers so that we could compare these with what we had learned of how they actually spent their time. We also compared the format and content of the minutes of key management committees before and after the arrival of general management. Finally, we collected performance indicator data for each English district for 1984–5, 1985–6 and 1986–7.

Thus the main focus of our study was on the perceptions of senior managers, medical and nursing staff as to 'what was going on'. Naturally we wanted to situate these beliefs in relation to other kinds of evidence and we also had a more pedestrian concern to avoid swallowing any 'tall tales'. We therefore developed a number of techniques for cross-checking. Most obviously, we cross-checked between individual respondents – if surgeon X said that general management in the district was a shambles and surgeon Y said it was going well we probed further in order to try to establish the source of the difference of view. Second, wherever possible we checked statements against documentary or statistical sources. Third, when we had drafted our preliminary findings we took them back to four of the health authorities in the sample and presented them to meetings of those we had talked to earlier. We also sought written comments from the individuals we had interviewed in the remaining authorities. In all this we were attempting to acknowledge the force of the arguments in favour of 'respondent validation' (Bloor, 1979; McKeganey and Bloor, 1981).

Finally, we developed an additional procedure which we hoped would clarify our thinking and at least marginally enhance the validity of our interpretations. In examining the question of the impact of general management we could hardly avoid posing the counterfactual question 'what would have happened if general management had not been introduced?' Some clarification of this counterfactual was necessary if we were to know which of the contemporary developments we observed could be attributed to general management and which would probably have arisen anyway (for an explanation of the notion of counterfactuals see Elster, 1978, pp. 175–221).

Our approach was as follows: first we assembled a small group of advisers, chosen on the basis that each possessed a mixture of academic and NHS experience. This panel was presented with a summary review of such research findings as there were concerning NHS management behaviour before the Griffiths Report. It was asked to modify and extend this summary picture in the light of group members' own experiences. Next, the panel was asked to project this pre-Griffiths situation into the post-Griffiths world – as if the Griffiths Report had not occurred but all the other variables were still in place. The panel's projection was then compared with a (previously unseen) account of the findings of our research. Finally, the plausibility of attributing differences between the panel's projection and our findings to general management was subject to critical discussions between the panel and the research team.

IMPLEMENTING GRIFFITHS: WHAT WORKED AND WHAT DIDN'T

The first step in the research was to record the views of NHS staff on the degrees to which certain features of general management appeared to them to be working in the ways that the 'official line' had suggested they should. The particular features on which we concentrated our questioning, observations and documentary analysis were:

- the setting up of new management structures within districts
- speed of decision-making and implementation (Griffiths had suggested that these could be improved)
- the clearer allocation of responsibilities to individual managers (again, Griffiths argued that this was both necessary and valuable)
- the usefulness of the Individual Performance Review (IPR) system (obviously linked to the previous feature)
- the development of greater responsiveness to the preferences of consumers of NHS services (Griffiths had claimed that the NHS was not close enough to its consumers)
- the use of management budgets and resource management as a key management tool (Griffiths had seen this as a key development)
- increased use of performance indicator data and other types of formal, comparative data which would enable managers to identify possible areas of weakness and strength relative to other, similar organisations.

One of the most striking features to emerge from our data is the way in which views on several of these issues show acute variation between different groups and levels of staff. For example, most of the nurses we spoke to thought that decisions were now taken more quickly (and generally approved of that) while most of the consultants thought the opposite. This suggests that the 'improvements' generated by general management are very unevenly distributed – indeed, in some cases they may be confined to the DGM, UGM and some directors of services, while most of the many other staff discharging management roles perceive little or no improvement. These patterns of light and shadow may be pointers for future management priorities.

In all the authorities studied there had been changes in formal organisational structures attendant upon the introduction of general management, and in most of them these changes had been substantial. Most general managers were keenly aware of their enhanced authority in matters of institutional design and many saw the immediate post-Griffiths changes as but the first steps in a continuing process of adjustment. In the first 18–24 months after appointment, general managers had usually felt obliged to spend a large slice of their time on structures and the appointments which set them in motion. Appropriate formal structures do not, by themselves, produce good decisions, but they can contribute to reducing overlap and delay, and to the grouping together of highly interdependent functions.

They can also carry a symbolic significance, for example when clear organisational equality is granted to a community function relative to an acute function. We encountered a great variety of local structures, but only isolated protest or criticism. In general the greater license given to DGMs to reorganise according to local circumstances seems to have been received with acceptance or even enthusiasm, at least by the majority of other managers. This generally positive conclusion is somewhat qualified by our findings concerning the ways in which hierarchical (i.e. structure-based) authority was sometimes being exercised (see below).

Senior managers were roughly equally divided on the question of the speed of decision-making and implementation. UGMs emerged as a group particularly likely to think acceleration had occurred, while district-based planners and administrators tended to be more sceptical. Consultants were the most pessimistic category – very few of them could see any speeding-up, while the great majority of nurses believed that decisions were being arrived at more quickly, giving as their main reason the elimination of one or more tiers in the nursing hierarchy.

Clearly, different staff were thinking about different kinds of decision. The optimistic nurses were usually referring to getting this or that done on the wards – routine operational adjustments. UGMs tended to cite minor works or changes in the deployment of nurses. Planners and administrators found the number of 'clearances' needed to get documents circulated and plans discussed were fewer than hitherto.

By contrast, both consultants and senior managers remained dissatisfied with the often slow handling of issues which involved going outside their own organisations. Much irritation was expressed by districts about regions and by regions about the DHSS (as it then was). The processing of major capital schemes was one particular focus of discontent, and public consultation procedures over closures and changes of use another. As one UGM summarised, there is still too much 'answerable to district, answerable to region'. Another UGM, who was particularly critical of the inflexibility of national terms and conditions of service, thought that while detailed decisions got taken more quickly, 'the total doesn't move very fast'. Analogies with steering giant oil tankers cropped up more than once. Several respondents – both managers and doctors – drew a distinction between speedier decisions (which they recognised were taking place) and more effective implementation (which they doubted). In addition to the alleged slowness of regions and the department they claimed that haste and lack of consultation meant that some decisions (e.g. in one case to convert a ward to five day status) came unstuck. Managers were then obliged to retreat and start again.

Most of our respondents thought that the introduction of general management had resulted in more precise allocations of personal responsibility. However, many of them also believed that this greater clarity did not yet extend very far down the hierarchy. Below UGM level, things became murky. Again, consultants were the most pessimistic group, a majority claiming that they could not see that the allocation of responsibilities between managers was any clearer at all.

IPR plans are one important way in which an individual's responsibilities can be clarified. In general we found that the IPR system was well received, with most respondents finding it fairly useful and some very useful indeed. Senior nurses and managers who were ex-nurses appeared the most enthusiastic. About half the UGMs, however, were critical. These managers experienced IPR as a rather top-down, time-consuming bureaucratic 'game'. Interestingly, performance related pay (PRP) was much less popular than IPR – even those who had benefited from merit pay 'bonuses' were uneasy at the way these might be interpreted by other staff. Our finding is that they were right to be apprehensive: consultants, nurses and more junior staff not infrequently passed cynical remarks about the motivation of senior managers who stood to benefit from PRP.

The development of greater consumer responsiveness is not an issue which emerged well from our research. A heavy majority of both the nurses and (particularly) the consultants we talked with thought that little or nothing of real significance was yet going on. There was widespread cynicism concerning what were seen as rhetorical or superficial gestures by management towards 'consumerism' while there remained glaring inadequacies in basic service provision. The consumer initiatives in various of our study districts were described as 'image building', 'lip service', 'glib', cosmetic' and even 'bullshit' (the last from a consultant member of a unit management group).

Of course, we also found individuals who were enthusiastic, and others who said they would have liked to do more if they were not bogged down in cost improvements and the latest priority initiative from region or Whitehall. We also found that some things were indeed happening – redecorated waiting areas, better appointments systems, training for receptionists, better hospital signs, floral duvets instead of traditional hospital bed linen, patients handbooks and numerous patient opinion surveys. These are all useful improvements but many staff found it hard to generate great enthusiasm for such 'frills' (a common term in our interviews) when basic standards of care were simultaneously under threat from cuts in staff and finance. One DGM candidly affirmed that his first and key IPR objective was to manage within the funds available, and that he had felt obliged to concentrate on this, possibly to the detriment of concern with the quality of care. In another district a UGM said that consumerism was 'like kicking fog – you could see it but you couldn't grasp it', and in any case finance was the priority issue. The overall message seemed to be that in many districts management was not yet succeeding in building a more consumer-responsive culture.

Our findings concerning the use of management budgeting (MB) and resource management (RM) are reported in greater detail elsewhere (Pollitt *et al.*, 1988). Very briefly, we found a few enthusiastic managers, but many cautious ones, and a handful of enthusiastic consultants but a large majority of determined sceptics. The sceptics included quite a number of consultants with extensive experience of MB – few of these had found the information they received to be particularly interesting or useful. It is important to recognise that these were not 'diehards', resistant to any consideration of resource constraints influencing medical practice. Most of the consultants we talked to were perfectly prepared to acknowledge the need for efficiency and economy, and a number of them made critical references to colleagues who, in their view, disregarded such criteria. RM was somewhat better regarded than MB (by both managers and consultants) but the difference was not overwhelming. Even those who believed that RM was the 'ultimate solution' (Director of Community Medicine) thought that it was foundering because it was being put to doctors in the wrong way.

Managers committed to RM in the long term spoke of 'doing the stone-dripping bit', of 'going very gently', and 'proceeding with caution'. Those with most experience were highly critical of the optimistic timetables sometimes floated by the NHS Management Board. Only two of the thirteen RGMs, DGMs and Scottish Health Board General Managers we interviewed seemed to be making MB/RM a key priority. Others took a much more detached stance. One DGM referred to RM as 'red herring' while a senior manager in a district said he preferred to let others make the mistakes. Elsewhere a DGM said that what he really needed was a reliable financial *control* system, which was not the same thing as management budgeting and need not constitute such a challenge to consultants.

Finally, we enquired into the use of comparative performance data. As far as performance indicators were concerned, our findings were in line with those of the major CASPE/King's Fund survey of 1987 (CASPE, 1988). Use of these indicators is now quite widespread, not least because most regions use them to raise questions with districts during the review process. However, use of PIs by DGMs and planning and finance staff appears to be far more frequent than use by medical or nursing staff. In so far as they are aware of them medical staff tend to question their accuracy (not always fairly, according to the CASPE research) and/or claim that they are not sufficiently detailed or sensitive to case mix to be of much use. 'We don't particularly trust them', as one consultant told us.

This and similar reactions naturally prompt the question of what performance data *are* used by medical staff. Here we found considerable differences from district to district and between specialties. Some departments were quite active, usually by adopting local medical audit, or by studying the Confidential Enquiry into Perioperative Deaths (CEPOD), or by taking up other intra-professional initiatives coming from the Royal Colleges. Others apparently do nothing, and we found quite a few individual consultants who remained cautious, or even downright hostile, towards the concept of peer review. Managers seemed powerless to do much about this. Clinical quality was still regarded as professional territory – or as one (rather pro-Griffiths) consultant put it, management stops at the consulting room door. On the whole post-Griffiths managers continued to accept this demarcation, although there were naturally occasional exceptions where the local cocktail of personalities was such that a respected manager was allowed at least to raise questions with the medical staff.

The Content of General Management Agendas

One of Griffiths' criticisms of the consensus management team concept was that decision-making was insufficiently proactive. It was seen as chiefly reactive and concerned with 'crisis management' and 'putting out fires'. At best, consensus management decisions merely endorsed the *status quo* and ensured it ran smoothly. At worst, difficult but necessary decisions were avoided. For Griffiths, general management implied a more strategic orientation and devolved responsibility for action. How far did general managers' agendas in our selected health authorities comply with this view?

In examining general management agendas, we were concerned with the following principal dimensions:

- the origins of agenda items and whether they were proactive or reactive
- the nature of the items: e.g. did they focus on financial control?
- National priorities? Local priorities? Specific local problems?

Management agendas comprised a number of inputs of varying significance. Local priorities jostled with national priorities for attention and looming over them all was the centrality of finance. At one level, the management agenda was long and complex. At another it was deceptively simple – keeping within budget. With 47 national priorities awaiting attention, the agenda was unmanageable for general managers. As one health authority chair remarked, 'in business if I had any more than 10 priorities my business was going down the drain'. The fact that many of the priorities clashed or appeared contradictory only added to the pressures on general managers. As a medical representative on a unit management board put it, it was an unacceptable situation for a manager to be told to cut waiting lists while at the same time to save money.

Without exception, general management agendas were dominated by financial considerations. The evidence from all our field sites overwhelmingly pointed in this direction. At best, general managers were obliged to balance a 'here and now' issue, that is not over-spending, with the achievement of the long term strategy, for example, dispersing patients from long-stay hospitals into the community. One UGM summed up the feeling of many general managers in stating that 'on occasion you could be forgiven for forgetting that there were actually patients in hospital'.

One UGM believed that general managers 'had been set up' to do financial management. 'The damage which has been wreaked in the last 12 months could not have been done without general managers on short term contracts'. The same UGM said that there had not been the same pressure from above on the issue of quality as on finance. No general managers had been sacked for lack of success on the quality front. For general managers whose priority was to survive beyond three years, together with the IPR system and short term contracts, there was little option but to accept a finance-driven agenda. Many accepted this reality with great regret and thought than an exclusive concentration on narrow efficiency issues carried real dangers for the long-term health of the organisation. Others were seen to possess, in the graphic phrase of a consultant geriatrician 'cash register eyeballs'. Clinicians were the most outspoken group in terms of criticising what appeared to them to be the dominant concern of general managers. According to one consultant, whereas previously issues might be discussed from the patient's angle they were now considered from a financial perspective.

Another concern of general managers was in shifting priorities in health services away from acute services. A district assistant director of finance/head of planning pointed to the mismatch between planning and resource expenditure. Even where community services were high on a general manager's agenda, there was a lack of success in switching resources from acute services. Management would renege on an agreed strategy and proceed to fund new consultant posts in the acute sector. Such incidents were common in the pre-Griffiths arrangements but were still occurring.

A key aspect of the Griffiths changes was that general managers had been singularly unsuccessful in confronting clinicians. As one senior official in the Scottish Home and Health Department put it, general managers 'are playing around the periphery'. Changes were taking place but mainly through attention to support services. Little attention was being given to clinical developments. Many general managers believed that Griffiths had grossly underestimated the power of consultants. One consultant, not untypically, believed that general management was 'unsympathetic to clinical matters'. Another consultant pointed out that 'since Griffiths we have had a lot more conflict. Clinical advice has been ignored, cast aside. The rift between the new general managers and the clinicians has become quite wide'. The same consultant pointed to a problem which had been identified by many of his colleagues both in this and other authorities, namely, that the idea than many clinicians would be interested in taking time-consuming management posts was 'one of the serious fallacies of Griffiths'.

Given the shape of managerial agendas, the extent to which general managers were seen, or saw themselves, as handmaidens of the government was often a matter of some concern. One UGM subscribed to the theory that their success as managers would be measured by their ability to keep the lid on conflict with other NHS professions and financial pressure. Several complained of being caught in a dilemma: namely, on the one hand, not ignoring the harsh realities of having to stay within budget while, on the other, devoting sufficient time to the long-term objectives set out in district plans. Moreover, there was a fear that involvement in a controversial issue like competitive tendering could damage a good manager's credibility with certain staff groups and make it more difficult to secure progress in other areas. As one UGM saw it, there was a problem of general managers at one level not being supported by those at other levels. Managers' efforts to build up trust and credibility could be undermined if the goalposts were constantly shifted by other levels. Allied to this concern was a sense that such pressures could not be entirely ignored, since success in general management would be determined by attention to national/regional concerns and not by advancing services locally.

Managerial agendas were virtually pre-determined by an overriding concern in central government with fiscal matters and, in particular, with 'balancing the books'. Coupled with IPRs and short-term contracts, general managers faced overwhelming pressures to conform to and accept a narrow, finance-driven agenda. For many managers, their immediate objective was to secure their future and have their contracts renewed. General managers spent a lot of their time reacting to short-term political imperatives.

These pressures seemed at odds with the Griffiths prescription for managers who would think and act proactively. While strategic objectives did figure among general managers' objectives they were not high on their list of priorities and were driven out by a need to deal with more pressing issues.

The Impact of Hierarchy

In this section we are concerned with the hierarchy of management relationships stretching from Management Board to unit level and with the relationship of this hierarchy to the medical profession. Griffiths urged the creation of a strong central management body committed to pushing responsibility down the line – 'to the point where action can be taken effectively' (NHS Management Inquiry, 1983). Managers were also expected to exercise a new authority. In spite of this commitment to delegation, other pressures (e.g. the desire for financial control at the centre) were making for a highly centralised system of management. The study produced evidence on the Supervisory Board-Management Board relationship, Management Board-region relationship, the region-district relationship and the district-unit relationship. In addition, it is necessary to consider whether hierarchically determined relationships are influencing clinicians. In Scotland there was no Management Board but there was a Policy Board. There was also no regional tier, only 'areas'.

Little evidence was collected pertaining to the *Supervisory Board*. This is hardly surprising since it met only on rare occasions. According to one Management Board member the low profile of the Supervisory Board is perfectly acceptable since it existed to act only as an 'umbrella against political fallout in many cases'. In Scotland the Policy Board met on equally rare occasions. Neither the Supervisory Board nor the Scottish Policy Board showed any signs of producing explicit, limited sets of policy priorities, or even clear statements of common values.

Our research in the regions uncovered a consistent view to the effect that the *Management Board* did not provide a strong central management influence on the organisation. 'There is no cohesion to what it does,' said one regional officer. At region, senior officers said that one to one contacts with individual Management Board members on specific issues were generally successful, but complained that no one seemed to be pulling the work of the Management Board together. One officer claimed region had constantly to ask 'where the strategic objectives were'. Respondents in the regions pointed to the detailed financial instructions which the Management Board continually issued as evidence of its confused sense of purpose.

Another regional officer regarded the Management Board as the key weakness in the general management structure. He blamed the lack of NHS trained managers at the Management Board's disposal for its poor performance. According to the same person 'the centre hasn't got its act together, it's not based on realism'. However, the Management Board also recorded some successes. The most notable of these was Performance Related Pay which was running after only 18 months. Nevertheless, we concluded that the Management Board was not delivering a corporate vision for transmission through the NHS hierarchy. In his Audit Commission lecture delivered in June 1991, Sir Roy Griffiths expressed his disappointment over the way the Supervisory Board and Management Board had developed. While both 'were absolutely correct in concept' they were 'half-hearted in their implementation. Major policy issues were left uncovered. There was no attempt to establish objectives at the centre and no concentration on outcomes' (Griffiths, 1991, p. 12).

In six out of nine English districts there was a consistent view among district officers and clinicians that *regions* adopted an overbearing posture with too much detailed interference. At the same time regional officers were accused of talking on a different level of assumptions than that current at district level. Region was therefore both a 'paternalistic and distant body'.

All categories of respondent accused regions of adopting a high-handed approach to policy. As one UGM put it when discussing the management of development monies, people would become disillusioned with her if she constantly had to tell them 'sorry chaps they've shifted the goalposts again'.

A strong feeling prevailed that regions undermined authority in the districts. In one region in particular officers in the districts complained about the level of detailed intervention going on. Regional officers were accused of failing to realise that requests for monitoring information generated considerable costs in terms of management resources. Several managers questioned the region's capacity effectively to intervene in detail. 'Region tries to meddle in affairs of detail which are beyond it's capacity for understanding'. Our evidence confirms the conclusions drawn by another research team (Stewart and Dopson, 1987).

We now move on to *district-unit* relations. On the whole UGMs said they enjoyed a greater authority and autonomy of decision making. Yet the evidence also suggests that the basis of these claims is questionable. UGMs in certain districts under financial strain complained about the contributions which were demanded of them by district to help meet the overspend problem. One UGM argued that since UGMs were the budget holders it was they rather than district officers who should be allocating contributions to savings packages. It was noticeable that in these circumstances clinicians consistently questioned the autonomy of UGMs. Two UGMs, one a recruit from the private sector the other a consultant, were frustrated with the propensity for district functional hierarchies to cut across their management of the unit.

In general, workable relations had been established between authorities and their units over respective responsibilities. However, the research did reveal a well-founded dilemma over 'contesting loyalties'. UGMs are clearly not wholly sure as to where their primary loyalty should lie – with the unit or the district/board. A consultant in a UGM post referred to the political game he played on behalf of the unit on the District Management Board. Another UGM pointed out that the conflict of loyalties undermined the capacity of the District Management Board to take a corporate view.

Only in one case did we discover an outright conflict between a UGM and a DGM. In this case the DGM had justified intervention in a series of matters on the basis that staff looked to district as the only legitimate source of authority. This was not a view backed up by interviews with doctors and nurses in the unit concerned. A number of other UGMs did acknowledge that the DGM or RGM had the right to deal directly with the clinicians in their unit.

Changes in the post-Griffiths manager's status had not in general resulted in a restructuring of the relationships between managers and doctors As one unit officer put it when asked how doctors had reacted to Griffiths, 'consultants are all right as long as it doesn't bother them'. At unit level where the relationship between managers and clinicians is perhaps most crucial, there was a widely held view amongst the consultants and nurses that UGMs had not found any substantial new authority. The opinion expressed by the chairman of the medical executive committee in one district that his colleagues still saw 'administrators as people who got in the way' summed up the dominant view amongst doctors. One consultant claimed that at unit level executive authority counted for little. Another saw UGMs as being able to act dictatorially on unimportant matters but lacking the 'clout' on issues of substance. He added that 'unfortunately the doctor always has the public's sympathy'.

In one district the UGMs even found it difficult to find a consultant willing to represent his colleagues in dealings with management. One consultant who had previously acted up as UGM thought that general managers could exploit the role of 'second-favourite' given the unlikely event of doctors actually agreeing. Another consultant in a different district believed that since consultants 'rarely spoke with one voice nothing happened unless a manager made it'.

Differences Between Authorities

Our prediction of finding substantial differences between authorities was fulfilled, but our expectation that this would be related to measurable differences in the tightness of resource constraints was not. For example, in one district which had always been far below its RAWP target (and looked like remaining so) the DGM insisted that there was no shortage of funds, and his claim was born out at least to the extent that complaints about resource constraints were less common in that district than in several others. By contrast another district which had been on or around its RAWP target for some years was rife with bitterness over cuts and shortages.

In so far as we could find a general explanation of the differences between districts under general management, it seemed that many of these had evidently existed before general management. They had merely continued, or been amplified, under the new regime.

Thus in one district, manager/doctor relations were quite close and discussions over resourcing were usually systematic and largely free of acrimony. In this case, however, the new general manager had simply inherited a pre-Griffiths regime which, over the years, had built up these strengths. In two other cases where, 'objectively', resource pressures appeared to be less severe, consultants were uncooperative and highly critical of local management. Significantly, in neither case had there been any tradition of close mutual working before Griffiths. When relatively modest clashes occurred in districts like these they could easily escalate into a general confrontation between management and the medical profession. Paradoxically, therefore, general management probably tended to work better in those places where the previous system of consensus management had itself been relatively successful.

There were signs that this might also be true of our two Scottish health boards. Here general management had been introduced later than in England and was less firmly implanted. The deterioration of the resource climate which had been evident in England since the early 1980s was only just making itself manifest. General managers were therefore in even greater danger than in England of being branded by health authority staff as mere financial surgeons.

Finally, one tentative observation was that management/doctor relations had perhaps undergone the most marked changes in the two districts where the DGM had come from outside the NHS. The staff in these districts tended to explain this in terms of the new DGM feeling less bound by cultural assumptions specific to the NHS. For a honeymoon period, at least, they were able to innovate more freely. Furthermore, their previous careers outside the NHS may have afforded them some initial status in the eyes of the consultants, status which the doctors would not necessarily accord to 'just another administrator'. It should be emphasised, however, that this breathing space could be misused. Whilst the two examples in our study had used their 'innocence' creatively, there were contemporary cases elsewhere which resulted in 'outsider' general managers leaving the Service very quickly after colliding with local doctors or politicians.

A Changing Culture?

As we have already noted in Chapter 1, the concept of an organisational 'culture' is a subtle one. It has frequently been bruised by use in mechanistic or over-simple ways. In particular, there has been a recent tendency to regard 'culture' as something that top management can mould and remould at will. This assumption has been fashionable in business circles and has frequently influenced the language of those advocating general management in the NHS (see, for a fairly temperate example, Barbour, 1989). Others, however, have argued that this approach is both conceptually and empirically over-ambitious (e.g. Meek, 1988; Pollitt, 1990, ch. 6; Turner, 1990, Introduction).

Our fieldwork yielded little suggestion that general managers were indulging in 'cultural management' as a conscious process. Nor had general managers succeeded in convincing most consultants that they should defer to a new management-led culture. No new set of 'key values' were in evidence – rather there was plenty of evidence of the old NHS 'tribalism', with each professional group displaying its own particular attitudes and priorities. Doctors still held to a predominantly 'diplomatic' view of the role of management – that it was the principal duty of managers to oil the wheels and seek out compromises between the various groups and interests comprising the service (Harrison, 1988a, ch. 3). What is more many if not most of the managers we interviewed did not themselves expect doctors to change. The model of a proactive management, setting goals, implementing plans for their achievement, and monitoring progress remained a vision rather than a reality. Reactive management remained the day-to-day norm, though now the reactions were as often to some centrally-inspired 'initiative' as to medical or nursing pressures.

In other respects, however, there was some movement. Most groups, including doctors, perceived themselves, and others, to be more managerially conscious than in the late 1970s or early 1980s. Yet as some respondents pointed out, this may have been as much a product of the financial climate as a specific effect of general management.

We also detected a sense of increased urgency, or pace, which did seem to flow from general managers. This was hard to pin down to specific examples, but it was widely believed nonetheless. Furthermore, Griffiths-model management did seem to have had quite an impact outside the medical domain. Among the administrators and nurses there were many who had accepted the 'message' and who acknowledged general management as a legitimate driving force. In the professional groups, however, this acceptance had seldom spread more than one or two rungs down the hierarchy.

ANALYSIS OF FINDINGS

Strategies for administrative and managerial reform in government and the public services may be classified according to a broad threefold taxonomy (Siedentopft, 1982, p. xv). First, there are *fiscal* strategies, which seek to reduce expenditure and costs while maintaining public services at roughly pre-existing levels. Within the NHS the cost improvement programme was intended to be such a strategy. Second, there are *structural* approaches, which 'seek to raise the productivity of public services without increasing costs. They concentrate on structural arrangements, decision-making, operating processes and the professionalisation of public agencies' (Siedentopft, 1982, p. xv). Siedentopft uses the term 'structural' to denote the range of relationships, processes and institutional arrangements that characterise organisations. Cultural features are also embraced by this category. Finally, there are *programme* approaches, which seek to adjust the quality and quantity of services delivered. Programme changes may result in the reduction (or increase) of the range or quality of publicly provided services. Privatisation is an example.

Utilising Siedentopft's taxonomy, the Griffiths Report adopted a predominantly structural approach. Unlike previous reorganisations, a conscious distinction was made between the means and ends of change. For instance, it was clear that the creation of a new body such as the NHS Management Board was not to be regarded as an end in itself. This approach is in contrast to the 1974 NHS reorganisation which placed considerable emphasis on administrative hierarchy and boundaries. Innovation in organisational design was, in Griffiths' view, only justified on the grounds that it would facilitate cultural change in the management of the NHS. The explicit focus on manager-doctor relations is indicative of the Griffiths management inquiry's rejection of attempts to represent the problems facing the NHS in a one-dimensional picture composed of 'boxes and charts'. That wholesale cultural change was being demanded by Griffiths was apparent to at least some of those interviewed. As one DGM, not in our sample, explained:

> The role of senior management has therefore less to do with taking decisions in the conventional sense than it has with fashioning a direction for the organisation; this will include a concern with developing a style of management (e.g. by delegation downward, systematic rational decision-making), in changing the characteristics of the organisation (e.g. by developing a responsiveness to individual patient need) and ensuring that there are effective mechanisms for policy and priority formulation, for implementation, and for monitoring and control of performance. (Liddell, 1988, p. 156)

In the authorities we studied this vision of senior management was not being realised, or at best only in a piecemeal and incremental fashion.

The gap between the Griffiths model of professional management and the untidier reality of the district health authorities in our sample could be explained in several different ways. One possibility is that the NHS was not trying hard enough – that the model was right but that there was more to do before it could be implemented. Another is that the model itself was flawed. For example, it could contain internal contradictions. Or it may inadequately have modelled the organisational dynamics of the NHS: perhaps the 'diplomatic' model reflected in many of our interviews captures something very basic in the way the NHS needs to be organised, something which was not given sufficient recognition in the original Griffiths analysis.

Some of those involved clearly took the view that the Griffiths model was right, but that it needed more time, effort and resources. For example, 'Griffiths is a very long process. The programmes I'm working with won't come to fruition until 1993' (UGM quoted in Strong and Robinson, 1988, p. 82). We certainly met quite a few managers who thought that, given another three to five years, information and budgeting systems would be in place which would allow them to behave in a way that approximated much more closely to the model of the systematically rational professional manager. Furthermore, the history of implementation studies warns us that many innovatory programmes falter at first, but, if they survive at all, are then modified and become much more effective as the organisations concerned move up the learning curve (Sabatier, 1986, p. 318). Those who take this view will no doubt take comfort from the considerable further strengthening of management so clearly intended by the white paper, *Working for patients*, a theme to which we return in Chapter 6.

Although we accept that further Griffiths-derived improvements are in the pipeline, and that it is still too early to essay any final judgements on the report's impact, we also wish to suggest that the Griffiths model itself is inadequate. [We would also point out that Griffiths himself, in evidence to a Parliamentary Select Committee, delivered the opinion that significant improvements should be visible within three years – that is by the beginning of our fieldwork period]. Our main critique is based on an identification of certain tensions internal to the Griffiths model plus an assessment of particular structural features of the NHS which we believe will continue to limit the likely impact of Griffiths-type structural reforms.

To begin with, there is a sense in which managerialism on the Griffiths model is founded on distrust, while the consensus mode of working is only possible on a basis of trust (Hunter, 1984, p. 94). The Griffiths model demands proof of performance – performance indicators, IPR targets, performance reviews of RHAs and DHAs and so on. Explicit objective setting and the generation of quantitative and/or dated targets is fundamental to this approach. Individuals and authorities are called to answer if they do not produce according to plan. This philosophy is given particularly sharp expression in the arrangements for general managers themselves to be employed on limited-term contracts. A degree of competitiveness is to be welcomed. By contrast consensus management and beyond that the whole diplomatic collaborative culture of the pre-Griffiths NHS is founded on trust. Relatively autonomous groups come together out of functional necessity, negotiate solutions which represent acceptable compromises between their several interests, and promise to deliver their part of the deal. To transform such a system into one in which identifiable individuals have to take personal responsibility for quantified targets is to shine a strong, harsh light onto processes of intricate political bargaining which may require degrees of flexibility, creative ambiguity and even downright secrecy in order to function most efficiently. This may be no bad thing, but it does cast doubt on the claim Griffiths made to be able to preserve the good features (unidentified) of the consensus management system alongside the new model.

A second, and more serious problem with the Griffiths model was its failure to offer a convincing analysis of the relationship between the business of running the NHS and the workings of the political system in which the Service is set. The NHS is a major, and highly popular public institution. It generates a never-ending stream of issues of local or national political interest. Underpaid 'angels' (nurses or ambulance staff); new wonder treatments; lengthening waiting lists; doctors with controversial diagnostic approaches to children who are suspected of having been sexually abused; other children who are kept waiting for treatment for life-threatening conditions because of staff shortages; scandalous conditions in long-stay geriatric or mental hospitals – the list is endless. Ministers have seldom been able to resist the pressures to intervene when one of these issues blows up, and there is no obvious reason to expect that they will exert greater self-restraint in the future. Neither at national nor at local level can a clear and stable line be drawn between 'political' decisions and 'management' decisions (Harrison 1982, p. 388). From 1985 to 1989 the part of the NHS closest to this volatile political process was that same part which Griffiths had designed to be the fount of consistency and steadiness in the longer term – the Management Board. Yet this Board conspicuously lacked constitutional protections or guarantees of independence – indeed, to have given it such would have required the kind of legislation which the promoters of Griffiths had foresworn in the name of rapid action. So there was an unresolved tension here, and one which the circumstances of resignation of the first Board chairman indicated to be far from purely 'academic'.

The third difficulty with the Griffiths model may be the most intractable. The proposed cultural revolution was posited on the existence of some tolerably clear objectives. Without them, the planning priorities and targets to which managers gear themselves, their career prospects and their merit pay bonuses all become merely arbitrary. If the political system cannot generate a set of ordered and reasonably compact objectives then either the NHS must continue to do without them or they must be invented internally, presumably by managers themselves. The problems with the latter solution are obvious: priorities generated in this way would lack democratic legitimacy and would not necessarily command the confidence of the main funding body – central government. Alternatively, it might be argued that the priorities against which NHS performance should be judged should be generated in a devolved manner, by district or regional health authorities. Yet such an approach would have additional drawbacks. First, it could lead to even greater inconsistencies than exist at present in scope or quality of service between one part of the country and another, inconsistencies which an increasingly mobile and well-informed citizenry would presumably find hard to understand or tolerate. Second, so long as health authorities remain appointed bodies the weakness in democratic legitimacy will persist. The Griffiths model does not address these matters. Instead it stands as an example of the kind of instrumental rationality in which profoundly political questions of priority and value are transposed into apparently scientific or technical issues (Habermas, 1971; Alvesson, 1987, ch. 7).

In the Griffiths Report managers are implicitly instructed to identify and apply standard techniques for dealing with NHS problems. Yet managers were acutely aware that the very act of defining problems in the NHS is a highly contested business. In classic or 'scientific' management theory the manager applies the correct technique to encourage employees to work harder. This raises productivity and success is reflected in higher output and profits. Workers are rewarded with higher wages and managers with a sense of professional accomplishment. But the targets facing managers are notoriously difficult to define and agree. NHS managers work in an arena where a profuse and unstable range of values and priorities must be taken account of. Success is a concept that has multiple meanings for different groups of actors. The Griffiths model seems to view the manager as a technician whose practice consists in applying the principles derived from management science to the problems of his/her organisation. In contrast, the *art* of management cannot be reduced to a set of simple explicit rules. In a setting like the NHS where there are multiple definitions of a problem and an abundance of often contradictory objectives, managers had in the past become more sensitive to the phenomena of uncertainty and ambiguity. In its adherence to a different theory of management, the Griffiths report was flawed.

There are consequences of such failure of analysis. Without clear objectives, *effectiveness* cannot be measured and therefore cannot function as one of the main criteria for organisational performance. Thus the kind of performance assessment envisaged within managerialism begins to slide towards a lop-sided emphasis on narrower notions of *efficiency* and *economy*. Several of the DGMs we interviewed were well aware of this problem. This slide is accelerated by the easier availability of input and process (rather than outcome) data. It has also been accentuated by the Conservative government's strong ideological predilection for reducing public expenditure (Pollitt, 1986).

Without objectives it is also very hard to discuss the kind of *programme* (as opposed to structural) reforms which might ease some of the pressures on the NHS. Business managers may ask 'what business should we be in?', but without guiding objectives it is hard for health authorities and NHS managers to do the same. The aims and purposes of the NHS remain grand, but vague. Explicit discussions of possible programme changes are both fractious and rare – even putting ancilliary services out to competitive tender has proven a long drawn-out wrangle, costly in senior management time.

Finally, our research has pointed towards the pervasive importance of two structural features of the NHS. Subsequent chapters return to these. The first of these is medical autonomy. The power of the medical profession has formed a central theme in the massive literature on health services organisation. Even among professions, doctors are unusual in the scope of their autonomy. In the NHS hospital consultants can, broadly speaking, admit whichever patients they choose, treat them in whatever way they wish, discharge them when they see fit, and leave it to others to sort out the resource and staffing consequences of these 'clinical' decisions. They cannot be instructed to alter any of these decisions by a manager, and the Griffiths reforms did nothing to alter this. It is even harder for consultants to commit their own colleagues to particular courses of action – the autonomy of the individual consultant has been the stumbling block to deals concluded both at national and local levels (Harrison, 1988a; Harrison *et al.*, 1989).

Both managers and consultants repeatedly testified to their awareness of this autonomy. 'It's like having production managers who aren't responsible to the general manager', said one district Director of Finance. A DGM in another, unhappy district complained that certain consultants were 'even worse than before' and that there was clinician resistance to general management 'across the board'. Most districts did not seem quite so tense, but in one there had been an explosion of consultant anger when cuts had to be made, and in yet another senior managers told us that in their view the participation of consultants in general management would dissolve if any attempt was made to close more beds. In two districts the chairmen of medical staff committees told us in almost identical terms that they and their consultant colleagues were certainly not accountable to the local health authority or its managers. More generally, the limited progress reported above in respect of new budgeting systems and consumerist schemes both had a great deal to do with consultant hostility or indifference.

Many consultants thus continue to maintain a semi-detached relationship with NHS management. In his studies of the implementation process Sabatier (1986) has demonstrated the importance of basing reforms on sound causal assumptions. In particular he has emphasised the jurisdiction component within such assumptions – to what extent are implementing agencies given jurisdiction over the organisational linkages vital for the achievement of the proposed reforms? In these terms the Griffiths model again appears deficient. General managers were not given sufficient fresh authority to do more than make very cautious, incremental progress towards harnessing consultants to management objectives. With respect to this group (though not to others) the frontier of control shifted only slightly in favour of management (Harrison, 1988a).

The second structural feature which has limited the implementation of Griffiths is the fiscal situation of the NHS. The marginally constrained ability of doctors to commit resources becomes even more problematic in a situation where central government is determined to restrain overall expenditure, yet both the demand for and the supply of health care are increasing. On the demand side there has been a growth in the size of the elderly population plus a more general rise in public expectations. On the supply side many NHS districts have experienced increasing surgical productivity – consultants treating more patients per unit of time – and while this usually lowers unit costs it increases total costs. This is not the place to go into the details of NHS financing (see King's Fund Institute, 1988) but it is essential to appreciate the interactions between the recent financial traumas and Griffiths-style management.

Two very widespread features of these interactions emerged from our fieldwork. First, most general managers acknowledged that, since 1986, an enormous slice of their time had been taken up with short-term financial manoeuvring. This had knock-on effects on how much time they were able to spend on other tasks such as encouraging greater consumer responsiveness, monitoring clinical quality or making strategic plans. Second, the constant search for economies meant that in the minds of many NHS staff general managers became closely associated with 'government cuts'. This in turn seems to have had an unfortunate effect on general managers' credibility as standard bearers for a positive new management culture. Many consultants told us that in their view money dominated general management. One medical staff committee chair – by no means anti-Griffiths – was convinced that general managers would implement cost restraints or get sacked. Another medical committee chair said his general manager was busy looking after his own security and commented, 'performance indicators – they mean savings'. Several UGMs acknowledged that staying within financial targets was the crucial thing. One explained that there were few quantifiable criteria for measuring his performance, but one of them was efficiency savings -- this was how he expected general managers would be judged. In yet another district the DGM told us that his personal agenda and that of other senior officers was at present totally dominated by finance.

Finally, financial stringency had undermined what might otherwise have been one instrument general managers could have used to persuade consultants to pay more attention to management concerns. DGMs could seldom offer 'sweeteners' (e.g. new staff or equipment) to motivate not-very-interested clinicians. In one district where the DGM had been very successful in persuading a number of consultants to take up management posts, several senior officers expressed the view that, if cuts had to be implemented (this was a district where the new general hospital was still expanding) consultant support would quickly collapse. In sum, financial stringency has cast a shadow over the Griffiths vision of a general manager-led cultural revolution.

Our final conclusion is, therefore, that implementation of the Griffiths model has been handicapped by tensions and limitations which were inherent in the original report, by flawed understanding of the management problem in the NHS and by wider developments (the failure of government to set clear priorities plus the deteriorating financial situation) which were beyond its remit. Despite this, its impact has been considerable, especially among managers and administrators themselves, and also with nurses. We would hesitate, however, to describe this as a major cultural shift: the diversity of NHS subcultures ('tribalism') remains, and the Griffiths model has not yet become dominant. In the words of a Unit General Manager: 'It has been a partially funded palace revolution, not a thorough-going, fully-funded management revolution'.

In Chapter 6, we comment on whether the changes being implemented in the NHS following *Working for Patients* promise to complete the management revolution which, if not started by the Griffiths inquiry, certainly got going in earnest as a consequence.

CHAPTER 4

A Review of NHS Management Research, 1985–90

PREVIEW

The purpose of this chapter is twofold. First, we wish to validate and extend our own findings by identifying points of agreement with other researchers. Second, where other studies have produced results which in some way confront our own findings we are obliged to try to explain why a difference has occurred. The extent to which we can undertake these operations is limited. It is quite apparent that the aims, scale and scope of research into general management require clarification. A brief summary is presented below by way of a pre-condition to drawing comparison between substantive research findings including our own.

AIMS, SCALE AND SCOPE OF THE NHS MANAGEMENT RESEARCH COMMUNITY

Under variously funded initiatives the academic community produced a total of 23 empirically grounded studies of management in the NHS between 1985 and 1990. In addition, the Association of Community Health Councils for England and Wales, and the Confederation of Health Service Employees (COHSE) also published the results of their own research.

Referring to Table 4.1, the first point to make is that the scale of research projects ranged from Pindar's interviews with five general managers (Pindar, 1986) to our own study which involved 339 interviews conducted in nine English Districts and three Regions, two Scottish Health Boards, and including local authorities, community health councils, trade unions and central government. Clearly the scale of our study was a necessary consequence of our more ambitious aims. Pindar, in contrast, was concerned to produce a record of early impressions of general management.

Table 4.1 Empirical research in the NHS: 1985–90

AUTHOR(S) AND PUBLICATION DATE	FIELDWORK	SCALE AND SCOPE	METHODS AND SOURCES
ALLEN (1986)	1985	72 DGMS	Interview pilots, Questionnaire
COE (1985)	1985	11 Regions	Documents (formal organisation structures)
CANDLIN (1989)	1985–6	Child health services in 1 DHA	Interviews
SMITH (1987)	1985–7	56 UGMs	Questionnaire
STEWART (1989), GABBAY & STEWART (1987), GABBAY & WILLIAMS (1987, 1989), DOPSON & GABBAY (1987)	1985–7	20 DGMs & their networks	Interviews, Observation, Documents
STRONG & ROBINSON (1988a, 1988b, 1990), ROBINSON & STRONG (1987), ROBINSON et al.(1989)	1985–3	7 Districts, plus all DHAs in England and Wales	Interviews, Observation, Questionnaire
CHANTLER (1988)	1985–3	Study of 1 teaching hospital	Observation
PINDAR (1986)	1986	5 General Managers	Interviews (attributable)
SCRIVENS (1988a, 1988b, 1988c)	1986–7	155 DGMs	Questionnaire (open-ended)

Table 4.1 (Continued)

AUTHOR(S) AND PUBLICATION DATE	FIELDWORK	SCALE AND SCOPE	METHODS AND SOURCES
GLENNERSTER & OWENS (1986, 1990) OWENS & GLENNERSTER (1988)	1986–8	1 Region, detailed study in 4 districts	Participant observation, Interviews
PETTIGREW *et al.* (1988, 1989a, 1989b) McKEE & PETTIGREW (1988, 1989) McKEE (1988) FERLIE & PETTIGREW (1988, 1989, 1990)	1986–9	10 Districts in 8 Regions	Documents, Interviews, Observation
SCARFE (1987)	1987	50 staff in 1 District	Interviews
JENKINS *et al.* (1987, 1988) BARDSLEY (1988)	1987	16 Districts	Questionnaires, Interview
HARRISON AND SCHULZ (1988)	1987	Psychiatrists in 1 Region	Questionnaires
ASSOCIATION OF CHCs (1988)	1987	69 CHCs	Open-ended Questionnaire
CONFEDERATION OF HEALTH SERVICE EMPLOYEES (1987)	1987	85 respondents in 4 Regions	Interviews, Questionnaire

Table 4.1 (Continued)

AUTHOR(S) AND PUBLICATION DATE	FIELDWORK	SCALE AND SCOPE	METHODS AND SOURCES
BANYARD (1988a, 1988b, 1988c, 1988d)	1987–8	88 Units in 2 Regions	Interviews, Questionnaire
HARRISON et al. (1988, 1989a, 1989b, 1989c) POLLITT et al. (1988, 1989, 1990) MARNOCH et al. (1989)	1987–88	9 Districts in 3 Regions, 2 Scottish Health Boards	Interviews, Observation, Documents
FLYNN (1988)	1987–88	6 Districts and RHA in 1 Region	Interviews, Documents
HAYWOOD et al. (1989)	1987–88	8 Districts in 1 Region	Interviews, Documents
COOMBS AND COOPER (1990)	1988–90	10 Districts	Interviews, Documents, Observation
BUXTON et al. (1989, 1991)	1988–90	6 Resource Management Pilot Sites	Interviews, Documents, Observation
WILLIAMSON (1990)	1987–89	65 respondents in 12 Scottish Health Boards (senior management level)	Interviews
SYMES (1988)	1988	14 units in 14 Regions	Questionnaire

However, it is not just simply the scale of research which creates a problem for attempts at comparison. The NHS, as earlier chapters have shown, is a complex network of professional, managerial and client relationships. Where exactly the 'general management problem' is to be located remains a subject of debate. For example, can general management simply be understood as the actions and beliefs of general managers? Alternatively, should researchers self-consciously concentrate on service outputs or, if this is problematic, on the management of service providers, notably clinicians and nurses? Few researchers have attempted to address this problem in clear theoretical terms. Usually the focus of research is in some way determined by a mixture of expediency and incentives dictated by the funding agency. Readers are referred to the record of empirical inquiry summarised in Table 4.1 in assessing the validity of comparisons between our own research findings and those of others. A few general comments are in order.

A total of six studies focussed exclusively on DGMs, while one study concentrated solely on UGMs. Two studies concentrated on a single professional group (in both cases psychiatrists). Around half of the studies dealt with only one level in the NHS hierarchy. Williamson's (1990) study was concerned wholly with general management in Scotland. Five studies dealt with only one region and its associated districts. Four research teams were motivated to study a particular feature of the management process – resource management, information, performance indicators, and planning. Only three studies, including our own, actually purported to present conclusions on general management as a whole. Of these, the study by Strong and Robinson was located at district level, though with a tendency to emphasise general management from the perspective of nurse managers (Strong and Robinson, 1988a; 1988b; 1990). The research team (Pettigrew and colleagues) based at Warwick University was in many ways the closest in aims, scale and scope to our own study. With a similar desire to capture the totality of general management's impact, the Warwick team interviewed professionals and managers at Regional, District and Unit levels. In offering this brief overview of types of research, we are in no way passing judgement on the differing aims of other researchers.

We have discussed at length elsewhere the potential for tension that exists between those responsible for policy implementation and policy evaluators like ourselves (Pollitt *et al.*, 1990). 'Proving' that a programme of change is succeeding or failing is not really what policy research is about. In the case of general management in the NHS the complexity of institutional and cultural change was of an order to put off researchers whose instincts are to reduce the policy arena to a limited set of quantifiable variables. No real 'axiomatic' management principle has been officially endorsed at either an implicit or explicit level. There is little therefore upon which to hang research aimed at establishing linkages between supposedly critical variables – for example, an index of managerial toughness and waiting lists.

Almost all the research projects depended upon interview and data generated from questionnaires. Although many of the research reports attempted to quantify attitudes and beliefs regarding the impact of general management to a far greater extent than we chose to do, we are nevertheless attempting to compare data sets that are ultimately qualitative in character. Implicitly or explicitly, a number of studies relied upon ethnographic methods. At one extreme, Strong and Robinson present their findings in what amounts to a continuous narrative composed of fragments taken from interviews. For our own part, we chose to structure our interviews loosely according to a theoretical perspective derived inductively from the Griffiths agenda. Broadly speaking, we took four categories as delineating possible change attributable to the Griffiths initiative. The issues in these categories are all evident in the presentation and anlysis of our own research findings set out in Chapter 3. The four categories are:

- hierarchy
- managerial orientation
- evaluation of change and outcome
- orientation to the consumer.

Change is theorised in terms of Handy's typology of culture, the Fordist, post-Fordist characterisation of control and a Lukesian conceptualisation of power (see Chapter 1). Additionally, it may be useful to reiterate certain points made in Chapters 2 and 3 as a means of signalling the perspective from which we compare our own findings with those of other researchers.

Power in the NHS is exercised along three dimensions – first, 'observable conflict' where issues are the subject of open contest between interested groups; second, 'non-observable conflict' where one or more interested groups are coerced by another group occupying an elite position from contesting an issue; and third, 'latent conflict' where, subject to ideological and cultural domination by the dominant group in a society, a range of issues exists where those groups in potential conflict fail to recognise their own interest position. Managers may encounter either observable or non-observable conflict when they press home changes against the perceived interests of other managers, nurses, ancilliary staff and doctors. However, managers are themselves the subjects of power exercised by doctors through the third dimension. In this latter case doctors rather than managers are the authors of those ideas contributing to the dominant 'commonsense' view of the world of health care delivery.

Consistent with this diagnosis of power relations, NHS managers can be said to operate in a hybrid organisational culture. Managers dominate a version of Handy's role culture which is inhabited by other managers, nurses, administrative staff and ancillary workers. Unusually, however, this co-exists with a Handyian person culture occupied exclusively by the medical profession. A key feature of the traditional hybrid NHS culture is that political and managerial control operated at arm's length and in reaction to resource committing decisions taken by doctors.

The peculiar nature of the traditional NHS culture has meant that the centre, mindful of managerial limitations, has been wary of attempts at tightening control over resources. NHS managers have become central figures in a command structure which could, with suitable enhancement, take on characteristics of hierarchy, centralisation, conformity and control over effort and working methods associated with Fordism. However, the medical profession does not fit this model, and never has. In fact, the medical culture appears to be closer to a post-Fordist model – a flat, decentralised network of specialised and/or local units held together by contractual relationships within a broad strategic plan. One distinguished interpreter of organisational life even goes as far as to cite the hospital, dominated as it is by doctors, as a model for big business to copy in the next century (Drucker, 1988).

Hierarchy

The Griffiths reforms were supposed to produce a clearly defined hierarchy of control extending from the minister down to the service providers. At first sight, this indicates a close adherence on the part of the Griffiths reforms to a version of Fordism. Yet a textual analysis of the Griffiths Report reveals a considerable degree of ambiguity about its proposed direction with respect to the manipulation of hierarchical relationships as a mechanism for exercising control. Indeed, the Report also employs what could pass as post-Fordist language in stating the need to push decision-making down to where it could be of greatest consequence – a seeming recognition of the knowledge-person-based nature of health care and the need to design a flexible management style for harnessing specialists' energies.

The ambiguous nature of intended hierarchical change is implicit in the evidence collected by other researchers. The hierarchical arrangements associated with general management have attracted the attention of a number of researchers. Early evidence suggested that apart from a few cases of outright opposition, doctors were ambivalent to the introduction of general management (Scrivens, 1988b, Harrison and Schulz, 1988). This is in sharp contrast to the hostility expressed by the medical profession towards the market ideas contained in *Working for Patients* which were seen as 'political' in a way that the Griffiths changes were not. For instance, only 19% of Harrison and Schulz's sample of psychiatrists could see only negative effects associated with general management. The implications of the Griffiths Report for manager/clinician relations might have been expected to open up a conflict, with doctors launching a campaign to retain professional autonomy. In practice, doctors did not immediately feel either under threat or inspired by Griffiths. Administrators and clinicians chose to pursue a degree of instrumental collusion in their relationships. Collusion or deal-making was an activity vital to the traditional NHS organisation. Without collusion the hybrid organisation could not have worked. Significantly, evidence suggests that the Griffiths changes did not remove the attraction of collusion as a political strategy for achieving ends.

Since to a large extent they could observe safely from a distance, doctors were not noticeably nervous about the changes in hierarchical arrangements. For others this was not the case. Nurses were immediately affected by general management, at least at the senior level. For senior nurses general management often meant a loss of managerial responsibility. With budgetary responsibility for nursing passing from the Chief Nursing Officer to UGMs, it was clear that senior nurses had to find a new position in the NHS hierarchy. The COHSE survey indicates that 64% of nurse managers thought decisions passed them by following the introduction of general management (COHSE, 1987, pp. 1–10). A study of nursing and general management carried out by Owens and Glennerster lays stress on the reduced status of CNOs (Owens and Glennerster, 1990, pp. 83–102).

> The conception of the role has had to change. Leadership has had to move towards negotiation and influence rather than authority and control This is more problematic in a system like nursing, which is based on a militaristic model. (Owens and Glennerster, 1990, pp. 102)

At Unit or ward level we found that nurses often welcomed what they saw as devolved authority. Owens and Glennerster also make reference to this positive response.

On a positive note Williamson, Banyard and Flynn have all provided evidence suggesting that greater clarity of responsibility has been achieved in the NHS through the introduction of the general management hierarchy (Williamson, 1990, Banyard, 1988a and Flynn, 1988). Banyard concluded that there was greater clarity at Unit level as to where responsibility lay on most issues but especially in respect of budgeting. There was also greater scope for developing unit policies, and communications had improved. Williamson notes that decision-making under general management seemed to be quicker and generally sharper. Chief officers felt they were in a stronger position to take decisions on their own where responsibility was clear. However, Williamson, like ourselves, also collected evidence suggesting that the new hierarchical arrangements in the NHS only speeded up decision making over small and medium scale issues. He, too, encountered the view that quicker decision making was not necessarily better decision making.

The ambiguous nature of grass roots hierarchical change was compounded by what went on at the centre. Surprisingly, researchers have paid comparatively little attention to the NHS Supervisory Board and the NHS Management Board. On the one hand, general managers were appointed to fulfil leadership roles, with decision-making responsibility pushed down to the level where it mattered. Yet, at the same time, the centre has constantly strived to increase its control over resources. Owens and Glennerster recognise this problem.

> The DGMs themselves felt that the hierarchical controlling aspects of NHS organisation needed loosening up. There's too much control still resting at the top, and there was not enough delegation downwards, thus limiting their capacity to manage. 'We are swamped by different priorities being manufactured by the DHSS – the flavour of the month attitude.'   (Owens and Glennerster, 1990, p. 70)

We found a similar problem arising in the relationship between Region and District and District and Unit. Williamson's study of the NHS in Scotland again uncovered similar tensions (Williamson, 1990, p. 29). Particular complaints were made by DGMs regarding what they described as excessive financial monitoring, top-slicing and earmarking of budgets (Flynn, 1988, p. 90, Pettigrew *et al.*, 1989b, p. 24). At unit level Flynn's evidence shows UGMs attempting to cope with contradictory commitments to District imposed cost improvement programmes and service standards. Like ourselves, Flynn recognised the importance that the financial context in which general management was implemented has played in its impact. Flynn questions the extent to which the type of control being exercised between Region and District, and District and Unit can actually be attributed to changes associated with general management. Strong and Robinson succinctly sum up the dilemma facing GMs:

> Griffiths, then, for all its radicalism, was only a partial break with the past. There was now a chain of command which reached from the top to the bottom of the organisation. There was also a new headquarters for staff with a potential flexibility to match the exigencies of local need

and form. But the service was still trapped, for general managers at least, within a national straight-jacket. Local initiative was frustrated by ministers, by civil servants, by supervisory management tiers, and by powerful professional bodies. Doctors still gave orders, nanny still knew best.   (Strong and Robinson, 1990, p. 164)

In response to a deteriorating ability or inclination to resource the NHS, the centre sent what has been interpreted as a shock wave signal to lighten command controls. Inevitably, given prevailing power relations and cultural barriers, this has had uneven consequences. A tougher role culture still had to coexist with a person culture dominated by doctors. Financial pressure caused managers to exercise authority with new vigour – but largely within the non-medical domain. The impact of tightened command control was therefore less important in organisational terms because of the frontier successfully maintained by doctors between themselves and managers. Though doctors like other groups found themselves constrained by a worsening resource position, they experienced this as a global climatic change rather than as a series of targeted management interventions.

Strong and Robinson argued that, in the absence of effective control, doctors will continue to dominate the NHS. Our own findings set out in Chapter 3 emphasised the importance of manager-clinician relations. It was clear from the very beginning that Griffiths had underplayed the importance of medical power. Pindar's interviews carried out in 1986 with five general managers are evidence that new appointees were well aware of the weak position they were in in relation to consultants (Pindar, 1986). One UGM is quoted by Pindar complaining that Griffiths had not redefined the role of consultants. This respondent argued that consultants still remained outside the employment of the district and yet the new style of management had to impinge on their activity if it was to make an impact. Another UGM admitted that his idea of the general management task involved everything but clinical activity.

The problem in establishing a hierarchy of command extending management into the clinical domain is reflected in the wide variation found in the formal structure of general manager/clinician relations observed by researchers, including ourselves. Scrivens discovered that the clinical directorate model, whereby a measure of managerial and budgetary responsibility would be devolved to senior consultants encouraged to manage their department, was the most favoured option amongst the 155 DGMs she surveyed (Scrivens, 1988b, pp. 27–31). Perhaps some surprise should be registered at this finding given the conservative bias that general managers had towards the traditional power-culture arrangement prevailing in the NHS. The clinical directorate model fits in well with the post-Fordist stress on decentralisation, and freedom from hierarchically imposed rules and authority. General managers were aware of the dilemma they faced in handing management responsibility to doctors without accompanying accountability. Often general managers had to offer incentives to secure involvement. The opposite strategy also had some supporters – Scrivens records four DGMs as expressing the view that they did not want doctors near operational management.

The Brunel study of resource management pilot sites also gives tacit support to the clinical directorate model. It is clear, however, that at least until 1989 most Units still operated a more traditional formal arrangement for linking doctors to the management process (Buxton *et al.*, 1989, p. 57). We should note that no central directive has ever been issued on the subject of organisational design relating to the interaction of clinicians and management. This is perhaps an indicator of the political uncertainty and caution surrounding manager-doctor relations even after the implementation of Griffiths.

The centrality of manager-doctor power relationships is thus reflected in much of the empirical research. Nevertheless, controversy exists over the extent to which the medical profession makes the NHS an exception to the familiar models of organisational hierarchy. For instance, the Warwick team claim that the theme of manager-clinician relations has been exaggerated in importance. Based on work carried out on the development of services for AIDS sufferers in a London District, a historical process of re-negotiating of roles, responsibilities and power relations is described. The problem of managing resources in response to AIDS demonstrates for the Warwick team that a potential exists for managers to intervene in 'ascendancy' to doctors. This claim is qualified by an acknowledgement that in practice the realisation of this potential has been accomplished only where specific local circumstances prevail. In particular, they draw attention to the quality of local information on clinical activity and outcomes, the intensity of the 'medical arena' (an important indicator being the presence of a medical school and attendant power relations), the history of previous manager–clinician relations, an effective leadership structure for delivering the clinicians to the decision making process and the existence of a clinical peer review system. While not disagreeing with the suggestion of a link between these factors and the ability of general managers to take the lead, our research uncovered few instances of managers enjoying such a favourable coincidence of circumstances. The general managers in our study had been unsuccessful in engineering the type of ideal management environment described above.

This view is further confirmed by the findings of Strong and Robinson, who believe that Griffiths failed to recognise that the NHS was effectively run by doctors. The Strong and Robinson material provides a lengthy description of a post-Griffiths NHS where medical power and individualism still runs through the organisation in such a way as to make all other professions peripheral. Our explanation for the more optimistic account of manager-clinician relations presented by the Warwick team revolves around the concept of power they employed and partly around the fact that AIDS was new territory in which the medical profession had not yet been able to establish its 'defensive strength'. As we noted in Chapter 2, similar forces were at play in respect of some community care services, like mental handicap services, where no medical vested interests were at stake.

Doctors enjoy several specific advantages over other groups in the NHS. They alone control the processes of diagnosis, referral, admission and choice of therapy. They did enjoy (prior to April 1991) particularly advantageous contractual conditions along with control over entry to the profession, status (particularly within hospitals) and income (through merit awards). They maintain a monopoly of practice over a wide range of activities. Yet these advantages would not necessarily be obvious in everyday working relationships in the NHS. Much of the time doctors rely on the manipulation of the 'commonsense' or 'traditional' ideas that complete the third dimension of power in the NHS. The third dimension of power provides the armour which protects the concrete foundations of medical autonomy from managerialist encroachment. Consequently much of our own evidence may be related to the concept of latent conflict – those instances of potential but unrealisable conflicts of interest held in check by prevailing 'commonsense' appreciations of what is right or proper in everyday relationships.

The problem of analysing latent conflict is that one is trying to explain a hypothetical – why conflict has not arisen over a particular issue. Essentially the researcher is dealing with inaction – explicable in terms of power and culture – but nevertheless something which has failed to materialise in any tangible form. We are not, of course, arguing that all potential doctor-manager conflict was defused and contained within the third dimension. For example, one member of the Warwick team draws attention to observable conflict in the form of interprofessional disagreement. In her study of the closure of a psychiatric hospital, McKee (1988) traces the conflict over leadership. She argues that clinicians pursued objectives that corresponded to a much longer timescale than that recognised by management. Clinicians refused to fit into the Unit's line management structure and were unwilling to take decisions through the Unit Management Board. Managers in McKee's study thought their own line management had been tightened by Griffiths but that little impact had been made on the control of clinicians. This evidence is in itself very useful in describing the real as opposed to formal position of general managers in the organisation. However, that clinicians could remain apart from the hierarchy that embraced all other NHS professionals is indicative of the *type* of power they exercise – concrete advantages armoured by ideological dominance. This gave them a strong position on all three of Lukes' dimensions of power.

Where open conflict has occurred this seems to have had little causal connection with the hierarchical aspect of general management. We would question whether the cases of service development for AIDS and closure of the psychiatric hospital studied by the Warwick team were significantly influenced by the position of general managers in the hierarchy. The counterfactual should be posed: would things have turned out any differently without general management? Had the hierarchical position created for general managers by Griffiths allowed them to challenge the power of the medical profession, open observable conflict would have been expected to have occurred during the implementation stage. In actual fact, as noted above, the implementation stage of general management did not greatly trouble doctors. In sharp contrast, our own and other evidence draws attention to the observable conflict which took place between general managers and the nursing profession (Pindar, 1986; Strong and Robinson, 1988a; COHSE, 1987). We believe, therefore, that differences between our own findings and those of the Warwick team are partly a consequence of differing theoretical treatments of manager-clinician relations and partly a function of the precise topics under study. While observable conflict yields more readily to empirical observation we believe that the hybrid nature of the NHS organisational culture means that a Lukesian three dimensional analysis has significant advantages.

The argument that the centre has failed to mount a strategy for breaking down medical domination and instead relied upon crude financial pressure as a means of forcing general managers to intervene over the level of clinical activity finds some support in the Brunel team's reports (Buxton *et al.*, 1989, pp. 53–60; Packwood *et al.*, 1991). They point out that the centre has chosen not to coordinate the resource management initiative. The pilot sites resemble six local projects rather than a national initiative. General managers at pilot sites and elsewhere have been allowed to adopt an accommodating posture which has in turn allowed resource management to be contoured around existing relationships with clinicians rather than being promoted as a bridgehead for substantial change. It has never been quite clear what the pilot sites were for. The Brunel team argue that where advances have been made with clinical resource management it has often been due to managers successfully drawing clinicians' attention to external threats to the resources at their disposal. This supports our findings that financial pressure lies behind much of the observable change which has taken place in the management of the NHS. In these circumstances the resource management initiative – the objectives of which were never very precisely defined – is in danger of being treated as a protective device rather than a management tool for realising long-term quality of care objectives.

Managerial Orientation

NHS general managers obviously did not use the academic language of Fordism and post-Fordism to describe their expectations, but it is clear that Griffiths appealed to them as a source of liberation from the constraints imposed by the traditional model. Allen's interviews with a small group of general managers conducted in 1986 reveal that they expected to occupy a more 'thinking' role and be less bound up in political power struggles. These general managers aspired to a position whereby they could genuinely claim to be directing the NHS towards particular service targets and expressed an optimism over the influence they could expect to have on clinical performance (Allen, 1986).

As time passed early enthusiasm could not be sustained. For instance, although 10 out of 12 of the DGMs interviewed by Williamson described themselves as 'directive', 'inspirational', 'strategists' or 'change agents' little evidence was subsequently discovered to confirm these characteristics (Williamson, 1990, p. 7). Our own findings revealed scant evidence of general managers having freed themselves from the reactive position endured by their predecessors. We concluded that financial pressures had prevented a more proactive style of agenda setting from emerging. The need to find cost improvements through efficiency measures left little scope for strategic long-term thinking of the type apparently envisaged by Griffiths. Evidence collected by other researchers supports this conclusion. Flynn is perhaps the strongest proponent of the argument that financial pressures more than any other factors have orientated NHS managers into a particular role. In his study of what he terms 'cutback management' he quotes a DGM explaining how the process of budgeting and planning had remained the same, and only the context had changed, being commonly dominated by the necessity of avoiding deficits. Finance, it was claimed, 'skews decisions' (Flynn, 1988, p. 125).

We believe that general managers still react to pressures and demands as opposed to creating conditions that influence the performance of key actors. Nevertheless, attention should be paid to the Warwick research team's study of a DHA response to AIDS. When doctors involved in coping with the AIDS problem found they needed new resources, they had to enter the management domain. In this way AIDS was transformed from being a clinical problem into a subject that would require the intervention of the DGM. The Warwick team believe that they witnessed a DGM taking charge of the AIDS problem when that individual was responsible for putting the brakes on spending. In this situation financial pressure is conceived as an incentive for a general manager to take a lead position.

Our own position is more pessimistic. First, we believe there is the question of whether the blocking of expenditure is itself an indicator of proactive strategic thinking. Also the counterfactual question needs to be posed – would a consensus management team have responded to rising costs in a markedly different manner? Consequently, we find the Warwick team's evidence less than wholly convincing as an indicator of strategic thinking on the part of managers.

This interpretation is reinforced by the Birmingham University study which was focussed specifically on general managers and their efforts at achieving efficiency gains (Haywood, Monks and Webster, 1989, pp. 1–5). Their conclusion that 'efficiency' had not yet entered general managers' value system might at first sight contradict the emphasis that ours and other studies have placed on financial pressures. In actual fact their evidence is not out of line with our own findings. Haywood and his colleagues see general managers working in a world of ever-shortening timescales – the budget position at the end of the year is typically the horizon of the general managers' vision. Concepts of efficiency have to be accommodated within this perspective. On the same theme Flynn (1988) records general managers treating cost improvement programmes as an externally imposed nuisance. On the basis of our evidence we can agree with his argument that finance has become separated from service considerations. The implementation of the cost improvement programme whereby managers are given percentage cost cutting targets is seen by Haywood and his colleagues as an example of the centre's inability to deny itself the opportunity of using general managers to slowdown the rising cost of health care. Inevitably under these circumstances the cost improvement programmes became a blunt instrument of hierarchical financial control rather than providing a framework for general managers to develop proactive leadership styles. Efficiency is not yet fully a part of the organisational culture – rather it is an externally imposed pressure to which general managers react. The pursuit of 'efficiency' was taking place within the bounds of the traditional model that places clinical performance off limits as far as managers are concerned, just as was the case of pre-Griffiths.

In addition, there is little evidence of financial pressure being used successfully by the centre to move managers in a controlled fashion towards a particular agenda. Smith showed that UGMs found it hard to separate underfunded pay awards from cost improvement commitments (Smith, 1987). In more general terms Haywood and his colleagues found no correlation between RAWP position and the orientation and enthusiasm of general managers for efficiency measures (neither did we).

Responses were haphazard products local circumstances. Given these conditions we believe Pindar is correct to conclude that general managers are still trying to fulfill a highly sophisticated management role against an environment charged with politics and professional power struggles (Pindar, 1986).

The Management Board has achieved little impact in de-politicising the NHS. General managers see themselves positioned between politicians wanting greater control over costs and an aggressively independent medical profession. At the same time, mechanisms which can be construed as attempts to force general managers to focus on clinical performance are not working. IPR and short-term contracts, we found, were treated with some degree of cynicism by general managers. As early as 1986 Allen reported that general managers thought it would be subjective factors that determined their career prospects rather than their ability to meet a clear set of quantitative and qualitative targets (Allen, 1986). Banyard, although an optimist over certain aspects of general management, also reported that IPR and contracts were not key motivators (Banyard, 1988a). The management budgeting/resource management initiative has failed to facilitate the management reorientation intended by Griffiths. Coombs and Cooper observed two resource management models emerging (Coombs and Cooper, 1990). The first they describe as being owned by doctors. In this case patient information has been built in with a view to enabling clinical research to take place. The second model is owned by finance departments. In this instance clinical information is played down and cost control is the real focus. It remains to be seen which model will become dominant. In short the centre has failed to give a lead to general managers so as to encourage a proative stance on their part. Managerial orientation is taking neither the shape of the Fordist command model nor a post-Fordist clinical performance orientated model. Concerns remained largely traditional in spite of all the structural change associated with Griffiths.

Evaluation of Change and Outcome

In a typical post-Fordist organisation, managers need the ability to monitor the cost and quality of work being carried out under flexible contract-based relations. We believe that general managers have been handicapped in the job of evaluating change and outcomes by the lack of a resource management system and reliable measures of quality. The evidence presented by the researchers at Brunel suggests that resource management has been developed in the pilot sites and elsewhere with greater emphasis on cost as opposed to activity data (Buxton *et al.*, 1989, p. 61) They are cautious on the prospects for resource management systems being utilised for the purpose of clinical planning and review, given that so few clinicians have contributed to the defining and testing of the systems. At best, resource management systems were being used on two sites to construct aggregate unit and clinical directorate objectives (Buxton *et al.*, 1989, p. 54). Only one or two successes have been recorded in general managers getting data to individual consultants which related to their clinical performance. No evaluation system based on standard targets was emerging out of the resource management experiments. The Brunel team found that a mixture of formal and informal arrangements were rather fitfully emerging between general managers and clinicians for collaboration over the setting of objectives, priorities and plans. Service providers were not being made responsible for the resources they committed anywhere below directorate level. As a consequence, accountability tended to be formal rather than real. Those attempting to lead resource management developments were placing greater emphasis on accuracy of data rather than on principles of accountability and evaluation of performance. General managers were not linking resource management to the review process. Positive answers were not forthcoming when the Brunel researchers tried to find evidence of resource management being utilised to apportion resources to service providers according to priorities. We believe this evidence supports our argument that resource management is being developed in a state of organisational isolation instead of being used to provide an evaluative linkage between general managers and clinicians.

Griffiths envisaged management budgeting providing the means for general managers to analyse clinical inputs and outputs. Since resource management has not been properly developed, general managers have had little option but to concentrate on maintaining costs at the aggregate level. Under these circumstances it is not surprising that treasurers or financial directors are the group who see themselves as having the most to gain from the introduction of resource management. Clinicians do not, in general, think resource management is worthwhile as a tool for evaluation (Coombs and Cooper, 1990, p. 6). Flynn (1988) records that where general managers, under financial duress, have had to tackle clinical activity, their usual practice has been to close beds. Only through this crude form of intervention have they achieved any success in making clinicians think about the link between clinical practice and resources.

The concept of evaluation is being impoverished by the concentration on financial control. Incremental growth patterns may be broken down through a process of hierarchically imposed financial restraint, but certainly there is no evidence emerging from studies of general management to suggest that rational evaluation of outcomes is a task that managers are in a position to tackle. One of Flynn's respondents, a

Director of Finance, confirmed that, even zero-based budgeting remained an impossibility (Flynn, 1988, p. 96).

While structural change took place at the centre with the creation of the NHS Supervisory Board and Management Board, little positive help was forthcoming in identifying evaluative criteria for general managers. Strong and Robinson (1990) made reference to a speech by a member of the NHS Management Board which they describe as 'brisk and bullish'. This person set out the stall for performance indicators (PIs) in the NHS:

> the continued wide range of variation (in health service activity levels) poses a number of questions. We've standardised many of the inputs so people can't plead special factors. What we have to do is to lift everyone from the bottom quartile to the mid-point. For the first time, the PI package offers us a major diagnostic tool. PIs also enable us to target our enormous resources onto patients. We need to be exact about what we're doing; for example, for particular age groups, or for prevention . . . And – somewhere over the horizon – we need to develop measures of outcome.   (quoted in Strong and Robinson, 1990, p. 171)

The confident tone adopted by this member of the Management Board belies the reality of uncertainty and confusion over the use of PIs in the NHS. Glennerster and Owens also noted – as did a number of 'our' general managers – that the centre has failed to confirm a limited set of service targets as priorities for general managers (Glennerster and Owens, 1990, p. 70). In the absence of prioritised service targets it is hardly surprising that the extensive (400+) range of PIs available to general managers remain inconclusive guides to action. Rarely did we encounter general managers using PIs as a tool for evaluation. This finding is supported by the detailed study carried out by CASPE on PIs (CASPE, 1988). This was a comprehensive research effort which involved a sample of 750 managers. (The definition of 'manager' used embraced nurses and doctors as well as general managers). A substantial proportion of the managers claimed to have used performance indicators – 85% of DGMs, 58% of UGMs and 54% of nurses. The indicators most intensively referred to were in bed provision and manpower. However, few 'ordinary' clinicians consulted PIs. Only 25% of clinicians in the position of chairman of the Medical Advisory Committee or its equivalent had used PIs.

When CASPE examined managers' purpose in using PIs, the results were not out of line with our own findings. It appears that managers used PIs as supplementary confirmation when bidding for resources. PIs were occasionally used to clarify an issue. Some of CASPE's respondents expressed the view that all RHAs demanded of them was that they keep away from extreme PI values. A number of respondents were also critical of the 'statistical approach to performance', which concentrated on process ratios and failed to tell them how effective a treatment was (CASPE, 1987, p. 29, Strong and Robinson, 1990, pp. 170–3).

The lack of output measures is one symptom of the centre's inability to set a limited number of service priorities. PIs have become part of general managers' defensive armour rather than a basis for the evaluation of service outputs.

Consumer Orientation

The traditional NHS model depended on rationing output to a passive patient population. For some time, the reality of a more informed and critical patient population has created problems for NHS managers and clinicians. While consumerism was placed centre stage by the white paper, *Working for Patients*, Griffiths had in theory already injected a degree of consumer orientation upon which to build. Our study uncovered a great deal of cynicism regarding things like 'window-dressing', 'charm school training' and *ad hoc* market research. (For a more optimistic view see Chantler's account of events at Guy's Hospital [Chantler, 1988, p. 10–11]). The Templeton College team assert that DGMs have been attracted to versions of consumerism which do not necessitate their entering the clinical domain. Our own study revealed 'quality' and consumerism to be concepts pigeon-holed with a particular post in the organisation (usually held by a senior nurse) rather than something which had entered the mainstream of organisational culture. Strong and Robinson's respondents reacted cynically to the tendency for DGMs to off-load the consumer-relations job into the domain of nurse managers. They quote a District Medical Officer who (unusually) also held the post of Director of Quality:

> some of the nurses and quality terrify me! . . . I've been really shocked by some of the ones I've met. They haven't a clue. They thought it was all about dealing with patients' complaints . . . some of the ones I've met think the idea is to get quality printed on T-shirts! . . . To give it to nurses just sets up the whole problem all over again.   (quoted in Strong and Robinson, 1990)

Strong and Robinson conclude that consumer orientation, and in particular the emphasis on quality, is really no more than a political gesture with little real meaning. While some initiatives have been worthwhile, we believe that the evidence for the period 1985 to 1990 indicates that the context in which general management was implemented militated against an imaginative and purposeful consumer orientation emerging in the NHS. It remains to be seen whether changes associated with *Working for Patients* will realise consumerist principles more rigorously (Harrison *et al.*, 1989).

THEORETICAL QUESTIONS ARISING OUT OF EMPIRICAL RESEARCH ON MANAGEMENT IN THE NHS

Much of the empirical research carried out on management in the NHS proceeded from a perspective that denied elaborate theorisation. In the remainder of this chapter we set out a theoretical assessment of the management problem in the 1990s. Through the process of drawing comparisons between our own and other research findings we believe we can justifiably extend the empirical foundations of the theoretical discussion that follows in subsequent chapters.

At the outset of our research that we pointed out that it would be a novel exercise simply to discover what general managers did. Empirical research conducted over the past five years has much advanced our appreciation of the management arena in the NHS. The process of comparing research findings provides us with a stronger empirical base to advance theoretical propositions on the management task in the NHS. However, in taking an overview of the research effort on general management two main deficiencies have emerged.

First, none of the research teams satisfactorily resolved the methodological problem of contextualising 'local conditions' facing general managers. This is not a task that yields readily to quantitative analysis. Like ourselves, the Birmingham University team could draw no correlation between management orientation and resource provision levels. (The Birmingham project used RAWP position as a proxy indicator). Where research teams laid stress on local conditions, they inevitably were concerned with qualitative factors such as the 'intensity of the medical arena' or the 'quality of clinical information'. The possibilities for developing a model that contextualises the management task need to be explored. Such a model would require both quantitative and qualitative indicators representing the forces, constraints and 'states of the world' confronting general managers. Potentially this could help provide a stronger analytic basis for investigating the management task.

A second area that remains a problem is the research community's understanding of medical power and management. It seems clear that the power exercised by the medical profession is qualitatively different to that exercised by any other group in the NHS, including general managers. Leadership is about exercising an intellectual influence over the direction of change, always necessarily complemented by dominance over areas of substance. General managers are not in a position to assume leadership from the medical profession. The only counter-evidence relates to circumstances where a combination of factors, including financial stress, have collided to place general managers temporarily in charge of events. Even under these conditions doctors have been adept in inventing tactics to evade crisis management measures. Chantler, for instance, observes that Guy's Hospital managed in 1984 to increase throughput and spending *after* closing 100 beds (Chantler, 1988, p. 3). The Griffiths managerial package, consisting of hierarchical restructuring, management budgeting/resource management, individual performance review, short-term contracts and annual review, has failed to manoeuvre general managers into a position of dominance over decisive functions in the healthcare system. Empirical research has failed to identify any linear mechanism for bringing doctors into the management domain. At the same time wholescale cultural change remains illusory. General managers lack the intellectual influence to create a solidarity of interest with the medical profession over the direction of change. Empirical evidence collected by the various researchers suggests that the old method of bargaining and compromise towards a position of instrumental complicity is still favoured by general managers. Given the substance of medical power, it is unclear whether the evidence indicates that doctors are beyond managerial control *per se*, or whether it is the case that the Griffiths programme of reform has not worked. In the next chapter we pay closer attention to the vexed matter of medical power in the management of the NHS.

CHAPTER 5

Managing the NHS

It is our purpose in this penultimate chapter to bring together, with a view to explaining, the issues raised both by our own research findings (presented in Chapter 3) and those of other researchers (described in Chapter 4). In so doing, we hope to provide a robust analysis of contemporary NHS management as we move through the 1990s. Chapter 6 then looks to the future and assesses the likely implications of the changes arising from the NHS White Paper, *Working for Patients*, which were introduced in April 1991.

A number of key questions have shaped the foregoing account of NHS management. First, what has been the evolution and critical junctions of management in the Service over the past forty years or so? Second, has the reform agenda over the years, commencing in earnest in 1974 with the first major NHS reorganisation, simply altered the *style* of management or has it sought to change the *substance* of management? Third, has the conception of management been a consistent one over the years or has it varied, reflecting wider socio-political shifts? Fourth, has the model of management that has been propounded been perceived as an appropriate one in the context of health care services or has its perceived inappropriateness led to an absence of substantial change in the practice of management? In this chapter, we pull together the various strands in the story and offer an integrated account. A further key question underpins the discussion which follows: how far can the gap between aspiration and reality which has been described in Chapters 3 and 4 be explained by reference to the notions of, *inter alia*, power, culture and puzzlement/uncertainty introduced in Chapter 1?

In seeking to address these questions, the subsequent discussion concentrates on five issues. The most important is to clarify the nature of medical influence. Despite having referred in some detail to theories and concepts of power and puzzlement in Chapter 1, the commentary in Chapter 3 on our study of general management was much more general. In particular, we now need to assess whether medical influence is power (if so, what are the corresponding dependencies?); or authority (if so, how far does medical legitimacy in the minds of managers outweigh government legitimacy?); or both. Closely linked to this is the question of why such influence seems more established and pervasive in some districts than in others. Is it related to the managers or consultants as individuals, or is there a more 'structural' explanation? A third question is also closely linked; we have shown that post-Griffiths management is still essentially reactive in character, though the agenda to which managers react has changed in that it is now primarily government-imposed rather than professionally-imposed. How far has this changed the balance of consultant influence towards the defensive? Fourth, we have shown that there is variation amongst consultants both in their orientation towards management and in their attitude to peer review and audit. We need to examine how far attitudes on these matters are related, and, if so, whether directly or inversely.

Turning away from doctors, a fifth important question centres upon the 'implementation chasm' that we so frequently identified. It seems important to try to identify factors that ameliorate or exacerbate this situation. Finally, still an immediate, but rather broader, question: the inclusion in our study of a Scottish-English comparison offers a kind of controlled condition in which many potential variables are held constant. It is necessary to elucidate the lessons of this comparison.

In our analysis of our research findings in Chapter 3 we suggested that the introduction into the NHS of general management and associated developments during the 1980s had not led to substantial change in the practice of management, especially at the interface between management and medicine. Consultants, by and large, continued to maintain a semi-detached relationship with management, and financial issues dominated general managers' agendas and distracted them from management concerns. That is not to say that the changes have been negligible or have made no visible impact. They have led to changes, as we and others have noted, but not so far (i.e. end of 1980s) in respect of the 'big' issues which inspired the reforms in the first place. Although they did not target the medical profession in quite the same way as the changes in the 1980s sought to, it seems from the available evidence we have reviewed that earlier reforms in the 1970s had a similar fate. Presumably that is one reason why policy-makers continue to meddle with the NHS's structure and management. However, the problems or practices to which their ministrations are addressed seem remarkably resilient and, to date, largely impervious to the favoured weapons used to attack them.

It will not have escaped readers' attention that some of the findings from our study of general management seem rather more pessimistic – even negative – when set alongside those of others (see Chapter 4). In defence of our position, we would argue that quite apart from the methodological differences between studies, together with the choice of different locations where substantial variation may be apparent, a great deal depends on the interpretation placed upon observed phenomena as determinants of subsequent developments. It is quite conceivable, for instance, that the rundown and closure of long-stay hospitals in respect of those with a mental handicap or mental illness – a major thrust of government policy in England during the 1980s – would have occurred with or without general management since economic pressures and resource constraints would have combined to provide a sufficient stimulus for action. On the other hand, general management's contribution (or lack of) to implementing the policy cannot be entirely dismissed. For instance, Korman and Glennerster (1990), in their analysis of the closure of Darenth Park Hospital in London, argued that general management provided a sharper, crisper focus and avoided problematic issues becoming bogged down in committees or teams. We return to this issue later in the chapter.

A further complicating factor in assessing the impact of such changes is the influence of personal style. While general managers may have accorded to them a modest set of powers and structural freedoms not available to their predecessors, these could not provide any guarantee of successful performance in their application. So, while not in any way minimising the achievements or impact of general management, we believe both that a sense of historical perspective is necessary, and that there is a recognition that the styles and personal characteristics of individual general managers count. This is why we have located our study not merely in the well-defined ideological climate of the 1980s – notable for its unremitting hostility to public sector management, especially in its pre-1980s shape and form – and deification of private sector management, but in the context of the evolution of management in the NHS from its inception.

What such a perspective offers, apart from continuity of explanation, is the need to distinguish between claims made for a set of changes from evidence of their actual impact on outcomes. Many of the changes which have occurred since general management, like a concern with quality and standards, medical audit and review, speedier decision-making, would probably have taken place anyway, albeit with assistance from the reforms. At any rate, they cannot be entirely laid at the door marked 'general management'. As we noted in Chapters 3 and 4, the changes in the financial climate were at least as instrumental in bringing about these changes. The converse of this view is that many of the desired or intended changes remained, at the time of our study, to be realised: notably the shifting of the frontier between management and medicine. General management may be unable to deliver on these if the model is based on an inappropriate (or on no) understanding of the micro-political dynamics of the NHS. Indeed, this seems to have been a constant feature of all the management reforms from 1974 onwards (Hunter, 1988). Thompson (1990), too, notes that NHS managers have not been as well served by the findings of research as they might.

There are echoes of the above in the first of the extreme explanations offered in, and subsequently dismissed by the Introduction: management changes come and go but the Service continues in much the same way. We do not subscribe to this simplistic view. What is at issue takes us back to the discussion of power in Chapter 1. Is it the case that, quite apart from, and in addition to, micro-political factors, larger, and possibly unseen, forces are at work which have had a more substantive impact on events and on the dynamics of the NHS than reformers have allowed for? Does the third face of power offer a more convincing basis for explaining events in recent years than simply taking the management changes at face value? To answer this question, we need to examine more deeply the 'special position' of doctors not only in the NHS but in society more generally.

THE MANAGEMENT-MEDICINE INTERFACE

As Klein (1989, pp. 222–3) has observed, a continuing paradox of the NHS has been that 'it exercises least control over those who, in theory at least, exercise the greatest influence in determining the demand for health care'. Moreover, tightening the managerial grip on the NHS and its providers – a constant theme in government policy since at least the early 1970s – does not mean that those who are ostensibly being 'managed' remain passive objects of managers' desires. A limitation – one of many – of an orthodox 'top-down' view of policy formation and implementation is its inability to appreciate or even comprehend the power of those on the periphery to shape policy and its implementation. This essentially 'bottom-up' focus is the subject of Lipsky's (1980) work on 'street-level bureaucracy', of which the medical profession in particular is a powerful and possibly rather exceptional manifestation. The profession owes this power at least in part to its overall position and status in the social structure and the high esteem in which it continues to be held by the general public. But it is also the case, as we argued in Chapter 1, that doctors enjoy considerable discretion over their work. Not all of this freedom for manoeuvre stems from their professional status. A great deal of this discretionary freedom stems from the nature of the work they do, the uncertainties surrounding much of it, and the limited resources at their disposal to carry it out. As a consequence, managers are highly dependent upon doctors without being able to intervene extensively in the way work is performed. In this respect, the relationship is one of both mutual dependence and potential conflict. Its importance lies in the position of doctors as *de facto* policy-makers as a result of their discretionary role, with all that this implies for managers at higher levels in the organisation.

In accounting for the occasional dislocation between our assessment of the NHS management changes in the 1980s and parts of that offered by other researchers, an explanation lies in the absence of a good theory of public sector management. Such a theory would endeavour to take account of the micro- and macro-politics of public policy noted in preceding paragraphs and to embrace concepts like power, culture and uncertainty. Not only can this lacuna account for an inappropriate model of management being repeatedly applied to the NHS, which is not our principal concern here, but it has most likely contributed to interpretations of the changes which have their roots in a quite different perspective, namely a business management perspective (Gunn, 1989). Such a perspective takes an apolitical view of how organisations function and may sometimes confuse style with substance or appearance with reality. Similar notions underpin Hood's (1991) discussion of a group of ideas known as 'new public management' whose origins lie in public choice theory and in business-type managerialism which has swept through the public sector in many countries, including Britain.

In Barrett and McMahon's (1990) terms, the shift underway in the NHS, and one that has gathered pace in the late 1980s, is from 'welfare values to market forces'. We consider in the final chapter how far this shift is likely to go, its implications for managers and management, and some of the impediments likely to be encountered along the way. Our concern in this chapter is with how far these competing perspectives, one focusing on business models of management and the other on micro-political and power-dependence factors, allow us to interpret and explain developments in NHS management over the past decade or so. The adoption of these respective approaches may also go some way towards explaining the differing interpretations placed upon the changes by different researchers.

From our discussion of power, puzzlement and culture in Chapter 1, it is evident that merely imposing a particular model of management upon an existing structure offers no certainty of success. Implementation failure remains a distinct possibility. Indeed, if the intention behind the NHS management changes was in part to end, or at least weaken, the complicity between managers and doctors then the reformers will be disappointed by the evidence of our research which, as we have shown, suggests that such a shift has not occurred to any marked degree. We need to qualify this statement by noting the variations evident between our field sites. General management appears to have had a greater impact in some than in others. The precise nature of manager-doctor relationships varied between the health authorities/boards in our sample. In order to account plausibly for such differences a macro-theoretical approach (i.e. Lukes' third face of power) has to be supplemented by a micro-level approach where notions of power, culture and uncertainty become shaped, even tempered, by the interpersonal dynamics and other local contextual factors evident at such a level. We develop this point in the concluding section below.

The uncertainties all too evident in the policy and managerial environment in the NHS, many of them triggered by successive changes in structure and management, have resulted in attempts to forge new relationships between managers and doctors. These range from polarisation and stand-off between the two groups to commonality of purpose against a common foe. While some doctors blame managers for the problems and pressures shaping their working environment, others regard managers as potential allies and as unwitting victims of a politically and ideologically driven reform agenda. Far from managing change, managers are seen to be glorified administrators doing the bidding of ministers as their agents. Clearly, where precisely managers sit in the system will, as it were, have a bearing on where they stand. At unit level, managers who are in close operational contact with clinicians often perceive themselves to be in a different relationship from those managers at regional level where the pressures from the central department will be greater than from the medical profession and therefore demand a different response.

As we noted in Chapter 4, where there is a semblance of solidarity between managers and doctors it is for short-term tactical reasons to enable consultants to retain a favourable position or to enhance it. The new managed relationship between these groups is tenuous and may, therefore, be short-lived.

For many, the intention behind general management was to change the culture. In the words of one former Regional General Manager, 'Griffiths wants to change the culture. He is trying to do a very much bigger task than just appointing a general manager' (House of Commons Social Services Committee, 1984, p. 80). But if this was indeed the case, then it has occurred unevenly and in an unbalanced manner focussing on managers but leaving the medical profession and its core attributes and position virtually untouched. While the management culture has visibly shifted, there has been no concomitant shift on the medical side. General management has not even challenged the medical domain never mind having succeeded in making significant inroads into it. Doctors' training and career patterns remain unchanged with the consequence that their basic beliefs and attitudes remain largely intact. Mid or late career training in management for a small minority represents only a marginal shift and not the culture shift forecast. Hardly surprising, therefore, that management budgeting and its successor, resource management, have made only slow and tentative progress.

Although general management's introduction may have resulted in marked changes in the management culture throughout the NHS, it is not clear how deep these go or whether they amount to little more than a veneer concealing beliefs and attitudes of a more deep-seated variety which constitute an inheritance from many years of managers having been hospital or, more recently, health service administrators. A reluctance to challenge or confront consultants may reflect the limits of the culture change among managers. Moreover, even if it is conceded that the culture may have shifted among managers, their actual *powers* have not changed to the same degree. Nor have those of the medical profession changed or been substantially eroded. Therefore, the management-medicine interface cannot be said to have moved to any marked degree following the introduction of general management.

THE POWER OF THE MEDICAL PROFESSION

Earlier we noted the need to clarify the nature of medical influence and to ascertain whether it is an example of power or authority, or both. Our view is that elements of both are on display although they vary between districts for reasons hinted at above. These reasons are both structural and individual in origin. They are structural in the sense that a key feature of professions is the power they are granted by governments to set standards of performance and hold their members accountable for achieving these standards. These are deemed to be matters of self-regulation rather than external audit (Light and Levine, 1989). This has remained the position since the NHS was created. Even medical audit, a major component of the 1989 NHS reforms being implemented, is seen primarily as an intra-professional educational rather than a management tool. The medical profession effectively operates the process while managers look on from the sidelines.

At the root of this issue is the thorny and contested matter of clinical autonomy. As many observers have noted, the type of organisation found in the NHS, and the distribution of power and authority within it, is deeply affected by doctors' special relationship to their patients which is at the core of clinical autonomy. We have argued elsewhere (Harrison *et al.*, 1989, 40) that 'claims to clinical freedom on the part of doctors can be seen as resistance against control over health care providers'. Clinical autonomy is invoked almost reflexively as a kind of ritual posturing but with the solemn purpose of defending doctors' territory from invasion by managers. In essence, what divides the two groups is that doctors (excepting the specialty of public health medicine) subscribe to, and are motivated by, different sets of values and objectives from those of managers. The two sets of interests may coincide on occasion over specific issues but there is a general perception that the concern of managers with budgets, priorities and the health of whole populations across localities is different from that of doctors, which centres on individual patients, meeting individual need and on not allowing resource issues explicitly to intrude into or dominate clinical decisions (Boyd, 1979).

An important issue in doctor power, and well to the fore in recent years, is the degree of alignment of professional interests with the public interest. This has been particularly noticeable over claims of NHS 'underfunding' and over the reception given to the NHS reforms outlined in the 1989 white paper where the concerns voiced by the medical profession are virtually identical to those expressed by the general public. Little matter that the medical profession has deftly shifted its position, undergone a late conversion and is a staunch defender of an institution – the NHS – which large sections of the profession were fiercely opposed to in 1948. Profession and public amounts to a powerful coalition which the medical lobbies have skilfully built up and exploited. The government and their managerial spokesmen in the shape of the NHS Management Executive appear unconvincing by comparison when putting forward their case, regardless of its intrinsic merits or demerits.

But while the coalition may be a powerful one, there are cracks appearing in the facade which may be seen to strengthen the general manager's hand if he or she so chooses. Hints or this were evident in our sample districts. If the late 1980s through the 1990s is to be the decade of accountability in health care, with a concomitant stress on outcomes and quality of life, then such a movement, if it can be called one, poses a challenge to medical dominance and potentially strengthens the cause of general management.

Without pre-empting the discussion in Chapter 6, the reasons go beyond fiscal pressures, political ideology, demographic trends and medical advances, important though all of these are. In recent years, a more critical attitude has developed towards the role of doctors and their relationship with patients (ironically, an unintended consequence of the government's NHS reforms may be to obscure or blunt this emerging critique). While the relationship has traditionally been marked by a deferential and uncritical attitude on the part of the patient, service users have begun to express greater concern over issues like variability in clinical practice, excessive waiting times for treatment and uncommunicative personal styles. Of course, and with some justification, doctors will maintain that inadequate resources are responsible for such perversities. But the reasons go deeper.

What is not clear from the research is the extent to which these issues will now be successfully tackled and, in so doing, how far managers will mount an effective challenge to doctors. The challenge need not be a crude or overt one involving open conflict. Much may depend on how vociferous public opinion is on the issue. But, as we have noted, the public by and large supports the medical profession and shares both its diagnosis (insufficient resources) of, and prescription (more resources) for, present difficulties. If politicians are losing the argument in the public arena, for how long can they continue to do so? How far can they or will they push on with the changes in the teeth of such opposition? If people exit from the service and 'go private' rather than remain in the NHS and give voice to criticisms of poor performance then it may be that public pressure will become weaker and more fragmented. But the government is not powerless. It does have genuine grounds for raising issues about the present mix of management and medicine and whether there is too little of the former in relation to the latter. Mounting research evidence shows that medical practices and interventions are not always as efficacious as is assumed or claimed. Medicine is by its very nature exploitative and meddlesome and sometimes medical interventions cause more harm than good (Illich, 1977; Illich *et al.*, 1977). There are, as the College of Health and others have shown, wide variations between hospital doctors in the number of patients treated, the length of time patients stay in hospital, and the resources used in treatment (Ham 1988; Andersen and Mooney 1990). Of course, we are unable to state unequivocally that such variations give rise to inefficiencies. They could simply reflect different constraints in different contexts. But they do prompt questions and the need to give closer attention to variations.

Resource pressures have contributed to a questioning of medical freedom because of the expansion of opportunities for intervention and their resulting cost escalation. As advances in medical technology open up new opportunities for diagnosis and treatment, tighter resource constraints have simultaneously widened the gap between the actual and the possible. Thus interest in the issue of medical dominance has grown, even among clinicians. Reflecting on these developments, Hampton (1983, 1237) has argued that if the resources are not available to do all that is technically possible then medical care must be limited to what is of good value, 'and the medical profession will have to set opinion aside'. A consequence of this is a greater emphasis on the evaluation of medical technology. This means doctors becoming more involved in and committed to medical audit as well as assuming greater management responsibility to ensure that priorities are established and resources used effectively (i.e. the purpose of the resource management initiative). In other words, what is intended to happen is that doctors, having chosen to remain apart from the organisation (i.e. the NHS) of which they are a crucial part, principally because it suited them, and possibly their patients also, to remain in such a semi-detached position, may be obliged to enter management in order to preserve their privileges (or to limit their loss) and to prevent or neutralise the impact of those changes which particularly concern them.

Doctors may embrace 'the new managerialism' not because of any change in culture on their part but because it is the only means available to them of protecting, and possibly furthering, their interests. If management is no longer prepared to come to medicine (i.e. the 'diplomat' school of thought) then medicine must go to (or into) management. As long as management remained weak, doctors could afford to remain outside it. If the situation changes and management becomes more powerful, or is perceived to be so, one possible strategy for doctors will be to enter it. The issue then becomes one of who is incorporating whom. Will doctors assume the management mantle and desert their clinical peers, or will they seek to use their position as a way of protecting those interests (see Hunter, 1992)? The evidence from clinicians turned general managers, limited though it is, is that the former may obtain. In respect of clinical directors, anecdotal evidence suggests a reluctance to confront colleagues and a wish to protect medical interests (see Harrison, *et al.*, 1989, 44–5).

STRATEGIES FOR MANAGING DOCTORS

Many doctors have questioned whether they have anything to gain from taking a more active role in management. Some are simply ambivalent about the merits of such involvement. They foresee an ethical dilemma if they switch from being advocates of the individual patient to becoming managers of resources. The view that they have always functioned as managers of resources on an implicit basis if not an explicit one is uncomfortable to them and is resisted by many. Such concerns go to the heart of the relationship between doctors and managers and of specific initiatives like medical audit and resource management which are designed to change it. To what extent doctors have positively or negatively embraced these developments is arguable and certainly varies across the Service. But the point is that management is not an abstract notion and the dynamic interplay between managers and those who are managed will determine its ultimate shape and orientation and the purposes to which it is put. Management is not an end in itself but merely a means to an end.

Three broad strategies are available to doctors, managers and politicians seeking to promote efficiency and effectiveness in clinical care (Ham and Hunter, 1988). These may be arranged along a continuum from minimal to maximal involvement by external agents (i.e. managers) (see Table 5.1).

At the minimalist extreme, a strategy of self-help among doctors is encouraged (e.g. by the profession itself acting through the Royal Colleges and professional associations) to raise standards and improve quality of

Table 5.1 Strategies for managing clinical activity

CONTINUUM OF MANAGEMENT INTERVENTION		
MINIMAL		MAXIMAL
Raising Professional Standards	*Involving Doctors in Management*	*External Management Control of Doctors*
• Medical audit • Standards and guidelines • Accreditation	• Budgets for doctors • Resource management initiative • Doctor-managers	• Managing medical work • Changing doctors' contracts • Extending provider competition

Source Ham and Hunter (1988)

care. A second strategy is to seek to involve doctors in management by delegating budgeting responsibility to doctors and possibly by appointing doctors as managers or as surrogate-managers (e.g. clinical directors). This strategy seeks to blur the boundary between doctors and managers in an attempt to agree and make stick common (or shared) goals. A third strategy is to strengthen external management control of doctors by changing doctors' contracts and encouraging managers or other doctors (external review) to supervise medical work more closely.

Government policy over the past 20 years or so, when viewed alongside these three strategies, seems to come closest to the first and second with some elements of the third visible in the 1989 reforms (e.g. new GP and consultant contracts). Others, like provider competition, remain hesitant and vague. How far the third strategy will prevail is uncertain. We shall return to these issues in the next chapter. From the evidence of our research, most managers resisted a heavy-handed, confrontational management style when it came to their dealings with doctors, preferring a minimalist softly softly approach.

BACK TO THE FUTURE

If the authority of doctors is looking bruised as a result of general management and related reforms, their power remains largely intact. Only time will tell how far this will remain so but from what we know of manager-doctor relationships at a micro level it is possible to speculate on the likely turn of events. We make this claim despite the evidence from some of the research on NHS general management reviewed in Chapter 4 to suggest that on particular issues – an example being developments in the care of people with AIDS – managers appear to have made inroads into clinical freedom. Our view is that such incursions remain the exception for reasons given in Chapter 4. In the case of AIDS it is a fairly recent policy issue and area of professional specialisation and while the medical profession has certainly been successful in the early stages in accessing the resources set aside to support initiatives in this area, doctors are not as uniformly well organised here as they are in other specialties. Where the concentration of medical expertise on AIDS is greatest is understandably in those areas where the disease is a major issue in terms of the number of people affected. Moreover, whereas the medical profession in such areas may have laid claim to being the major stakeholder in service provision, there is now a widespread recognition that the problem is not primarily a medical one but a social one, and that what is needed in respect of people with AIDS is good community care rather than medical treatment in isolation (Beardshaw, Hunter and Taylor, 1990).

The example of AIDS demonstrates that it is necessary to look at each particular instance of medical dominance separately, since the factors involved are likely to vary from example to example. While the medical versus social care dichotomy is not unique to AIDS, it is fair to say that the professional response to, and colonisation of, this disease has not become as entrenched as in other more traditional and prestigious areas like heart disease, lung cancer and so on where the clinical grip is tighter.

In a top-down view of health policy, governments propose (or enact) and managers, in their capacity as agents of the centre, dispose (or react). However, given the notion of power-dependence which we introduced in Chapter 1, a top-down view of policy and management is naive and simplistic. Either managers and doctors will join forces to 'game the system' or, if managers become mere functionaries in the 'chain of command' from units up to the Secretary of State, then doctors will attempt to subvert or bypass the management structure. Some doctors, as mentioned earlier, may join it in the hope of negating its most feared consequences.

Some idea of the impact an interventionist style of management has on clinical activity can be gained by experience in the United States. Potentially significant for developments in the UK, despite numerous attempts to strengthen the micro-management of clinical work in the United States, they have failed to control costs and raise standards. Indeed, expenditure continues to rise sharply and quality appears to have fallen – or at least it remains widely suspect (Herzlinger, 1989). Any attempt to regulate clinical activity from the outside (the third strategy in Table 5.1) is likely to be both resented and resisted. Any moves towards introducing an overtly aggressive management style into the clinical field could therefore be both counterproductive and ultimately self-defeating.

Extending provider competition, as the NHS reforms seek to do (see Chapter 6), could appear to be a more attractive approach to changing clinical behaviour. Again, however, the experience in the United States illustrates how doctors, sometimes aided by managers, are frequently still able to circumvent controls over their work (Notman, *et al.*, 1987; Weiner, *et al.*, 1987; Caper, 1988). While 'managed competition', to borrow Enthoven's term, may seek to make inroads into clinical freedom, in the United States it appears to have had only limited and temporary success in containing costs and maintaining quality. For instance, Notman and his colleagues found in their study of the effects of DRGs on doctors that

> the physicians are finding ways to comply with the formal procedures associated with the new regulations while avoiding or minimising some of the unwelcome constraints it puts on their behaviour. They have found ways of getting around system constraints to continue to give their patients the medical care they feel is appropriate.

'Fitnessing the system' in this way seems a likely stratagem to be employed by clinicians in the UK, possibly aided and abetted by managers, particularly those in provider units whether NHS Trusts or directly managed units.

A major issue in the context of NHS management is the extent to which, if at all, the changes we and others have observed in management in the 1980s have begun substantively to redefine the manager-doctor boundary and realign the power-dependency relationship which we have portrayed. At the time of writing, the jury is out and the verdict unknown. But from our research, and that of others (if to a lesser degree) general management has not yet transformed the relationship between doctors and managers. There have been skirmishes at the margin but the core of the relationship remains untouched. Exceptions to this can be found in specific instances in particular localities but they are perhaps only exceptions which go to prove the rule and for which local circumstances and personalities, or the issue itself in the case of AIDS, may provide convincing explanations. No single theoretical framework can capture or explain all these sometimes local, contingent or idiosyncratic influences on behaviour. Indeed, many of them elude complete capture by researchers.

What the evidence from our own work and that from the US suggests is that developments aimed at encroaching upon doctors' territory risk stimulating a range of perverse behaviours directed towards circumventing the controls and regulations imposed by management. As Caper (1988) has noted, 'as fast as regulations and review protocols are written physicians learn to circumvent them, resenting the intrusion into their clinical autonomy'.

Why has our research on general management thrown up such issues so sharply while other work of a related nature has not done so to quite the same degree? We venture to suggest that the answer may lie in an absence of analysis of the data on the one hand, and a lack of theory to explain observed phenomena on the other. By employing concepts like power, culture and uncertainty we have focussed the analysis on the underlying political nature of management in the NHS. If other researchers have reached different conclusions from our own we would argue that a major reason lies in the inductive approach we have partially adopted in respect of generating theory and because our perspective has been informed by an approach which is drawn from political science. If we re-analysed the data collected by others using our theoretical and conceptual approach we might have reached different conclusions from those they presented (and vice versa). But we should not exaggerate the differences. There are many similarities in the conclusions reached by a number of studies, and where differences exist, as in the analysis of the AIDS example by Pettigrew and his colleagues, there are good reasons for this which do not seriously challenge our conception of the prevailing power relationships between doctors and managers within the NHS.

We have chosen to view the NHS as a political system in both macro and micro senses of the term. In this way, it becomes possible to analyse the political strategies and tactics which managers, doctors and other stakeholders employ to secure desired ends. It is necessary to keep both macro and micro perspectives in balance since the operation of power, as we saw in Chapter 1, comes in different guises and is evident at different levels. It may be evident in the foreground of action at a micro level but, more likely, it exists in the background at a macro level. Adopting such a twin-pronged perspective allows us to view organisations (whether the NHS as a whole or its constituent authorities) not as uniform, monolithic entities but as heterogeneous and highly variegated ones.

Organisational life in the NHS is made up of different and sometimes competing interests many of them, as Lipsky (1980) demonstrated in his study of frontline operators, possessing the power to further them. Sometimes, though not always, the power is conferred and therefore legitimised (as in the case of the medical profession); sometimes it is acquired as a result of particular expertise or positioning in the organisation (for example, the role of the casualty reception clerk, see Hughes 1989). Understanding the dynamics of organisational life within the NHS requires sensitivity to the multiplicity of actors, the interactions among them and the differential bargaining power at their disposal. All of these may result in conflicts of values and interests. These need not be played out at an overt level but may well condition the response of different stakeholders in the system to particular initiatives or changes.

Not all events can be explained by reference to political manoeuvring or, as we suggested in Chapter 1, to the influence of power, culture and uncertainty. This last notion is especially important in the context of doctors' discretionary role. Sometimes the key players in an activity are confronted with puzzlement or uncertainty as to what they should be doing and how they should be doing it. Heclo (1975), for instance, maintains that references to competing claims should not be taken to imply that all, or even the predominant feature of, social politics is conflict in the play of power. Because the issues faced in health care are so complex, the major difficulty may be not the exercise of power or political will but rather the determination of what that will is, or ought to be. In other words, the situation confronting managers and doctors may be less one of competing for power and more one of coping with uncertainty, or the 'possibly unwinnable dilemmas' of health policy.

In our field sites, while the power factor undoubtedly had a bearing on the processes observed, in particular the relationship between managers and health care professionals, perhaps more in evidence on particular occasions were the constraints and uncertainties surrounding decision-makers in a setting where there are no clear measures of output or performance. Output measures based on numbers of inpatient admissions or days of care are conceptually inadequate when what ought to be discussed is the tangible contribution made to people's health. As health service managers and providers frequently point out, it is extremely difficult, if not impossible, to say that additional input 'X' has led directly to improvement in health status 'Y'. Allied to this is the difficulty of actually knowing when an objective has been met. For example, what level of service provision constitutes an adequate level of care for elderly people? Or when is it possible to say that enough has been provided in the way of services for those with a mental disorder? Heclo expresses the dilemma succinctly: 'social politics arises because men [*sic*] disagree among themselves, but also because they do not know what to do or how to do it'. To this extent, decisions and policy *result* – they do not get *made*. Rivlin (1971) reaches a similar conclusion in her claim that social problems remain unsolved

> because we do not know how to do it . . . The difficulties do not primarily involve conflicts among different groups of people, although these exist. Rather, current social problems are difficult because they involve conflicts among objectives that almost everyone holds.

IMPLEMENTATION GAP

Our own research on the impact of general management, and that of most other researchers, has shown that the challenge confronting it has been tougher than perhaps even Griffiths had anticipated it would be. There are a number of areas where this has proved to be the case. We comment on four here, the first three of which have been dealt with at some length in earlier chapters. In the conclusions to this chapter we argue that some of these outstanding concerns long pre-date the Griffiths changes and therefore suggest something deeper about the operation of power, culture and uncertainty in the NHS.

Financial issues have proved dominant for general managers. A heavy concentration on these has prevented a more proactive, strategic orientation from emerging. In part, a continuing preoccupation with financial matters is evidence of the absence of managerial freedom in the NHS with the overbearing presence of the centre, in the shape of the Treasury and Department of Health (not to mention Parliament), never far away. The centre continues to set much of the agenda for general managers at a subnational level. The research evidence also reveals that developments in management budgeting and resource management have either failed or are proceeding fitfully in the absence of profound changes in the beliefs and attitudes held by the medical profession, and in the absence of new levers of influence held by managers. Fragile efforts to embed the resource management initiative (RMI) in selected pilot sites, and to engineer the culture shift demanded in the manager-consultant relationship, may now be threatened by the 1989 *Working for Patients* reforms with their unseemly stress on a rapid roll-out of the RMI across the NHS in advance of any real evidence that it works or of what has to happen to improve the chances of success. So, even in an area heralded by Griffiths to be of fundamental importance to the success of general management, progress has been faltering and remains highly problematic. We return to the issue in Chapter 6, where we speculate on its future in the light of the reforms.

A third area to which general management addressed itself was consumerism. Again, as was mentioned in Chapters 3 and 4, notwithstanding some useful progress in respect of quality of service and consumer issues, most of these attempts have proved to be of a superficial 'window dressing' variety. No real or lasting attempt has been made to involve users directly in choices about priorities or service design – even if managers had ideas as to how to go about securing such input.

Turning to our fourth area of implementation failure, our findings, as well as those of others, have also been critical of the failure of the general management and related reforms to implement changes in national policy long-heralded by government as a top priority. We were unable to identify much positive evidence of general management having been successful in engineering a shift in emphasis from inappropriate long-stay institutional (i.e. hospital or smaller unit) provision to community-based alternatives for the priority care groups, namely, people with a mental illness, mental or physical handicap, or who are elderly. Indeed, as we noted above, managers were, often at their own admission, preoccupied with other more pressing concerns. But the difficulties in implementing the long-sought-after shift in the configuration of priority care group services have a longer history. Implementation failure in the area of national policies goes back to the 1974 NHS reorganisation (see also Hunter and Wistow, 1987). One of the thrusts of an integrated structure and a stress on improved management was to facilitate coordinated decision-making in respect of health care and community health services. Disappointing progress was made as a result of these changes. While general management was not advocated as a specific response to such problems it was hoped that national policy priorities would receive more serious attention since general managers' performance would be judged against it. It proved to be a wildly optimistic and naive view of implementation in a complex public organisation.

Gunn (1978) has identified 10 preconditions to achieve perfect implementation which are helpful in explaining implementation failure. They are:

• that circumstances external to the implementing agency do not impose crippling constraints
• that adequate time and sufficient resources are made available to the programme
• that not only are there no constraints in terms of overall resources but also that, at each stage in the implementation process, the required combination of resources is actually available
• that the policy to be implemented is based upon a valid theory of cause and effect
• that the relationship between cause and effect is direct and that there are few, if any, intervening links
• that there is a single implementing agency which need not depend upon other agencies for success or, if other agencies must be involved, that the dependency relationships are minimal in number and importance
• that there is complete understanding of, and agreement upon, the objectives to be achieved; and that these conditions persist throughout the implementation process
• that in moving toward agreed objectives it is possible to specify, in complete detail and perfect sequence, the tasks to be performed by each participant
• that there is perfect communication among, and coordination of, the various elements or agencies involved in the programme
• that those in authority can demand and obtain perfect obedience.

Few, if indeed any, of these preconditions prevailed in the implementation of policy in respect of new forms of care for the priority groups. Certainly some proved more problematic than others, notably the presence of external circumstances, allegedly insufficient resources and time, the absence of a single implementing agency, and of agreement over objectives. General management may have been a vital component of securing progress towards successful implementation but could not compensate or substitute for deficiencies in other areas. As Gunn observes, 'when implementation involves, as it often does, innovation and the management of change, then there is a particularly high probability of suspicion, recalcitrance or outright resistance from affected individuals . . . ' (p. 175). As we noted, the NHS is made up of multiple groups and interests who do not necessarily share the policy goals emanating from higher levels in the organisation. Policy for the priority groups is a particularly acute example of such dynamics in action.

Implementation failure is not necessarily the fault of general management. Indeed, in some of our districts general managers struggled against all the odds to make progress. The fact they either failed or were only partially successful has less to do with general management *per se* than with the prevailing culture, resource context, organisational relationships (both intra- and inter-), uncertainties in the external environment and the power-dependencies among key groups of stakeholders. They conspired to act as a more powerful determinant of policy implementation than general management. Where successful progress was possible in particular local circumstances, the converse prevailed though instances of this were, given the complexities, understandably more rare.

A TALE OF TWO COUNTRIES

As we suggested at the start of this chapter, the Scottish-English comparison afforded by our research study throws into relief a number of issues. These have been documented more fully in Hunter and Williamson (1991).

The overriding impression gained from a comparison between Scotland and England is that in Scotland developments, which followed those in England, initially amounted to riding on the coat-tails of the English rather than choosing general management through an independent process because it was right for the health service in Scotland. Even at unit level, where there was early doubt about the introduction of general management, it was virtually a foregone conclusion that general management would be introduced at this level at some point. As a result, the introduction of general management in Scotland was for the first few years, including the period of our research, more about style and less about substance than has been evident in England.

Despite similarities and obvious common problems and constraints (many of them covered in Chapters 3 and 4) it is possible to point to a greater number of changes flowing from general management in England. Evidence for this comes, in particular, from the management-doctor relationship: developments with resource management and clinical directorates have developed apace in England in contrast to the virtual absence of activity in Scotland. In relation to consumerism and quality of service, both key concepts in the Griffiths Report as we have shown, there has been faster progress in England even if much of it has fallen short of expectations.

Perhaps a healthy scepticism is in order in view of some of the wilder claims made for general management which have been found wanting. But it is hard to avoid the impression that the position in Scotland has been more akin to a form of 'dynamic conservation' – an attempt to fight to stay in the same place – rather than a bold attempt to fashion a new and distinctive management style for the health service in Scotland. One general manager has put this down to a left-wing bias in Scottish public life (quoted in Delamothe, 1990, p. 655):

one always gets painted with a black brush if you're changing anything in the NHS in Glasgow and perhaps in Scotland generally where there tends to be a fairly left of centre trade union oriented attitude to life.

The general manager who uttered these words alludes to two levels of culture change: that relating to organisational culture within the NHS, and that relating to the wider socio-political culture prevailing in a country. In regard to the first level, whatever dynamic conservatism prevailed in England, the desire to change or 'break' the stable state within the NHS has proved greater.

At one level that of structural change there has been greater convergence between England and Scotland. Notable exceptions are primary care services. But if there is now less distinctiveness about the organisational furniture in Scotland, differences between the countries remain, though less visible to the casual observer. Explaining them is a difficult task.

The cult of managerialism which gripped the NHS in the 1980s certainly did so with more impact and effect in England than in Scotland. These developments, as we have noted in Chapters 3 and 4, coincided with, and to some extent were prompted by, growing financial pressures in the NHS. In the absence of acute fiscal pressures in Scotland, the NHS may have been protected from the full impact of the new managerialism which may have resulted in less emphasis on the need for general managers to make a quick impression by balancing budgets. Finance did not appear, on the evidence from our study, to be driving or dominating general managers' agendas in Scotland.

A deeper explanation for the differences may lie in the stronger, and more confident, public sector ethos prevailing in Scotland. Conceivably, it has succeeded in absorbing general management before it had time to change the culture. If this is so, then a comparison between the two countries is useful in demonstrating (a) how difficult it is to separate isolated changes from their overall socio-political context, and (b) the need to adopt a more realistic approach to the claims made for general management. The fact that general management may have made a more significant impact in England than in Scotland may have less to do with general management itself and more to do with the overall socio-political and cultural setting in which it has been played out. A comparative focus has therefore been useful in forcing us to widen the search for plausible explanations which go beyond the mechanics of general management or the behaviour of general managers. Just as wider cultural factors have helped the medical profession to retain a position of hgh social status and respect, so have they lead to general management and related reforms being viewed with greater suspicion in Scotland. Whether in time the NHS reforms will succeed in challenging this stance in Scotland is an empirical question which we cannot yet answer.

CONCLUSIONS

As we pointed out in Chapter 3, many of the concerns to which the Griffiths reforms were a direct response remain alive. There has been an absence of substantial change in the practice of NHS management with the result that issues like manager-doctor relationships, consumerism, and the shift in priorities towards traditionally deprived care groups continue to exercise the minds of managers with little evidence of successful responses to such matters having been found or, if found, widely applied. As readers will recall from our earlier discussion in Chapter 2, many of these issues have their origins in the pre-Griffiths NHS of the 1960s, 1970s and early 1980s. More than previous reorganisations, the Griffiths changes were a conscious attempt to move away from a 'boxes and charts' approach to organisational change to one which sought to disturb organisational processes and ultimately change the beliefs and values of NHS actors. While there has been limited evidence of process change, it is not startling and managers continue to be preoccupied with many of the concerns which dominated their agendas, or those of their predecessors, in the pre-Griffiths era. While the way in which the Griffiths changes were implemented may be partly responsible, we believe the real reasons lie in the flawed nature of the proposals themselves and the assumptions about rational management on which they were predicated (see Chapter 3).

By employing a theoretical perspective drawn from political science with notions of power, culture and puzzlement or uncertainty to the fore we hope we have been able to account for the relationship between doctors and managers and the problems over implementing policies within the NHS. Such a perspective also accounts for occasional variations between authorities/boards, between different groups of managers and doctors, and between different issues which, though giving rise from time to time to different coalitions of interests, or to changes in the balance of power between interests, do not pose a threat so fundamental as to demand a wholesale reassessment of the management-medicine interface.

Much of the variation to which we have pointed is a feature of local contextual circumstances – hence our stress on doctors' 'micro power' at street level. Our evidence leads us to argue for a more clearly articulated model of the locality to explain such difference. This is not the place to develop a model in detail but we offer a skeletal framework drawing on evidence from our research presented in Chapter 3 and on the reflections offered in this chapter.

In the preceding discussion we have pointed to the critical nature of the relationship locally between managers and doctors (GPs might also be included but we do not do so here). For the most part, it is a 'steady state' relationship that is governed by a set of structural features, such as the nature of the consultants' contract and the absence of managerial instruments for exerting power. But it is also the case that local variations may result in a different mix or balance in the relationship so that it diverges from the average or norm. Our research locations provided a number of instances to illustrate the point. We comment on four.

First, we found that the legacy of history and inherited features in a particular locality shaped the precise configuration of culture, power and uncertainty in respect of doctor-manager relations. In one location the historical position of numerous acute and prestigious specialties, coupled with their concentration on several sites, certainly made the management task more of a challenge than would have been (indeed, from evidence elsewhere, was) the case where such a high profile medical presence was either weaker or absent. In this particular location, other factors and influences combined to make the power of the doctors appear even greater. The management culture was weak at both a structural and personal level and resource pressures, though evident, were not so acute as to provide managers with the leverage over consultants which some had sought to acquire in other locations.

These issues lead on to the second factor which we call the skill factor. This is an important variable in the exercise of power. Some managers and doctors are able to use, or are more adept at using, the power resources available to them. Such competencies may lie more in the realm of 'softer' interpersonal, political skills than in the area of 'hard-nosed' task based skills emphasised by much current management development education (Hunter, 1990). All other things being equal, a skilful manager will achieve better than average influence over local consultants.

The resource issue mentioned above comprises our third variable. With the possible exception of our two Scottish locations, where resource pressures are visibly less acute than in England (see Hunter, 1982), our fieldwork in the other locations did not reveal the resource factor to be of direct or easily discernible importance. The evidence from our Scottish locations nevertheless showed it to be of importance because the position is different in the Scottish Health Service.

The fourth variable is put forward more tentatively. It refers to the number of major acute hospitals in a district or board. Where only one such hospital (i.e. a district general hospital) existed, there seemed to be closer and generally better manager-consultant relations. Where there were multiple major acute units, there was much more suspicion among consultants as managers were suspected of favouring particular sites or hospitals. Managers played a 'no win' game in these circumstances.

Of course, not all these variables would apply in each locality in equal measure. In order to describe the dynamics of a particular process or activity it would be necessary to identify both the variables at work and their intensity. Our argument is that the impact of management reforms (or, for that matter, any others) in the NHS cannot be fully understood unless both macro- and micro-perspectives are employed. It is the interaction between these, and the interaction between the variables described above at the micro level, that leads to a particular outcome or configuration of power, culture and uncertainty between the actors in a given locale.

In this chapter, we have highlighted the importance of locality and described the variables which can result in deviations from it. But it is not only local variables which can modify the dynamics or relationships between key factors. These can be shifted if national changes at a macro level are introduced. With the changes announced in *Working for Patients*, and enshrined in legislative form in the NHS and Community Care Act 1990, there is the prospect of such a shift. Indeed, that is their intention. They can be seen, in terms of historical continuity, as taking forward and building on many of the managerial changes introduced by the Griffiths reforms.

The consensus over the principles underlying the NHS does not constitute an iron law, and the politically negotiated order which binds the NHS together at the turn of the decade may require to be renegotiated as we move through the 1990s. Indeed, this looks likely to be the case as the 'most far-reaching changes in the history of the NHS', in the words of the former Secretary of State for Health, begin to bite. It is to these that we turn in Chapter 6.

Before doing so, a brief recap on our conclusions so far is in order. As this and earlier chapters have demonstrated, the Griffiths reforms have centred on shifting the management culture in the NHS in order to achieve three things: a Service that is managerially-driven rather than profession-led; one that is proactive rather than reactive in its management style; and a Service which is sensitive to user preferences. Not surprisingly, such a massive change of agenda has encountered problems and has succeeded only in part. Clinicians have not willingly given up their power since they believe it is not in their, or their patients', best interests to do so. They possess a monopoly of information over treatment options and maintain they are acting as patients' advocates. Managers, with some exceptions, have not sought to mount a full-frontal assault on clinicians' power base. At best they have sought to work through RMI and other incentive-based initiatives to modify clinician behaviour. More typically, managers have been reluctant to confront clinicians and have chosen instead to remain absorbed by familiar NHS preoccupations, notably financial constraints, waiting lists and the struggle to implement national priorities. The new NHS that is being shaped could hasten the revolution begun by Griffiths.

CHAPTER 6

Going to Market?

INTRODUCTION

It is inevitable that this final, future-oriented chapter should be more speculative than its predecessors. The task is to extend the fabric of our analysis of the recent past so as to clothe the present and near future. Despite voluminous conjecture, we necessarily possess only the most preliminary and fragmentary information about the working of the 'provider market'. Nevertheless, we are convinced that our chosen analytical tools remain relevant to the post-*Working for Patients* (*WfP*) NHS. The coming of a market can most certainly be analysed in terms of shifting power relationships and changes in organisational cultures.

We are not going to take up space with a detailed description of the *Working for Patients* arrangements. Such material is available elsewhere (for instance, the annexe to Harrison, Hunter and Pollitt, 1990) and some command of 'the facts' is therefore assumed in what follows.

Neither is it feasible to examine every facet of the *WfP* changes. Instead we will focus on the role of management, and in particular on the themes which have occupied most of the earlier part of this book. Thus we have divided the chapter into six main sub-sections. First, we return to the issue of hierarchy and enquire what kind of authority structure is likely to survive the advent of a quasi-market and a split between the functions of purchasing and provision. Second, we look again at the resource management programme, previously a limited number of pilot schemes but now said by many NHS managers to be an essential component of the new arrangements. Third, we examine the likely agendas of general managers in the mid and late 1990s. Fourth, we explore the new purchasing role of post-*WfP* DHAs and link this to the issue of public accountability. Fifth, we present a short analysis of the relationship of Community Health Councils to the new management structures. Sixth, before offering a brief conclusion, we reflect on changes in the relationship which has become so central to the development of the NHS over the last decade – that between managers and the medical profession.

HIERARCHY

We begin at the top, with the Policy Board and the Management Executive. The creation of these two bodies was said by the *WfP* white paper 'to introduce for the first time a clear and effective chain of management command running from Districts through regions to the Chief Executive, and from there to the Secretary of State' (Department of Health *et al.*, 1989, p. 13). On reflection it may be seen that this was rather a curious cuckoo in the nest of a provider market. Markets, of any kind, are not run by a single clear chain of command. On the contrary, in the words of one of the more profound recent analysts of command and market systems: 'a market system is a "spontaneous order" monitored by its feedbacks, it conflicts with a "rational order" shaped by targets' (Sartori, 1987, p. 400).

But if the notion of a command centre does not fit comfortably into the new world of an internal market, neither does it correspond to the traditional NHS culture described by pre-1983 research. This earlier pattern might be summarised as being one of local diversity modified by occasional bursts of regional or central paternalism and overlaid with an encompassing, but cumbersome and ineffective framework of bureaucratic planning. So how can the *WfP* prescription best be understood? Our inclination is to see it as an ill-fitting fragment of an alternative vision of the NHS. This alternative has never really got off the ground, though it has probably attracted some support from senior Department of Health officials and from a few, perhaps many, post-Griffiths NHS managers. It is a vision of a unified, hierarchically-managed NHS in which managers finally enjoy both the power and the information to abandon both the diplomat and the economiser roles and to become truly proactive. The Service would then be run through manager-set plans and targets which, for the first time, could be enforced. Both local political interference (from local authority members on health authorities) and medical recalcitrance would be much reduced by re-structuring and resource management (RM) so, at last, rational managers could manage. A 'chain of command' also has attractions for ministers in so far as it allows them to claim that, despite the introduction of market mechanisms, the requirements of full public accountability are met.

If we are even half correct about this interpretation, it represents a partly obscured alternative to, rather than a part of, the proposals for a provider market. This alternative is none other than the Fordist, or 'command' model introduced in Chapter 1. From this perspective the NHS is analogous to an integrated firm. A market, by contrast, produces not a central spine of command but diversity, innovation, local deals and solutions, a set of rival providers who make their own, competitive plans. The important distinctions are between purchasers and providers, not between levels in a hierarchy of command. And the mode of interaction between the constituent bodies within a marketised NHS is one of negotiation and contract monitoring, not 'command'.

Is the hierarchical 'command' model the only possible interpretation of the roles of the Policy Board and the NHS Executive? Clearly not. It is only one of a number of perspectives (or, more grandly, implicit models). In the private sector the 'command' approach favoured a centralised organisation run on hierarchical lines. The integrated firm operated through direct, command-type instructions to its constituent parts. These parts were divisions or departments – integral parts of the one unified organisation. The whole was held together by uniform regulations and by a master plan developed at or near the top and then promulgated down the hierarchy. In the public sector the same notions were reflected in a variety of forms. In the late 1960s and early 1970s there was a fashion for very large organisations which it was presumed could develop and implement strategic plans (Pollitt, 1985).

The 1974 reorganisation of the NHS was influenced by this trend. These giant bureaucracies had a number of similarities to the giant private sector corporations which were flourishing at the same time. During the Thatcherite '80s macro-planning went out of favour, partly because of its ideological association with socialism and partly because of the perceived planning failures of the preceding twenty years. In its place came a focus on tight financial disciplines and meso and micro-level controls of work volumes. It was a kind of re-born version of F. W. Taylor's scientific management, only this time mediated through computers and directed at white collar rather than blue collar workers (Pollitt, 1990a). This new emphasis affected the NHS as it did virtually every other part of the public sector. Performance indicators, manpower targets, Rayner scrutinies, cash planning, cost improvement programmes and Individual Performance Review were only some of its manifestations.

From the mid 1970s, however, a new organisational model was beginning to gain favour in the world of business. Before long it began to influence the public sector too. Characterised by high degrees of decentralisation and flexibility, this was the 'post-Fordist' model described in Chapter 1 and elaborated in subsequent chapters. Here the huge unified or 'integrated' organisation is fragmented into a larger number of operational units which are then loosely co-ordinated by a central organisation. The latter remains free of the detail of operational management and need not become enmeshed in the intricacies of rival production technologies – indeed the post-Fordist process has sometimes been referred to as the 'externalisation of production'. Nevertheless, the centre retains control. This it accomplishes not by means of a hierarchy issuing instructions, but rather through a mixture of sub-contracting, franchising, networking and partnership arrangements with whichever seem to be the most efficient and innovative producer organisations (Mulgen, 1988; Zuboff, 1988).

If this begins to sound like some versions of the post-*WfP* purchaser/provider split, that is no coincidence. The idea of a provider market is very much in line with the post-Fordist model of control:

> Thus the movement within the public sector towards contracting out, devolved financial management (in the health service and education, administrative decentralisation etc.) needs to be read as something made possible by the transformation of the technology of control as much as the outcome of particular political strategies pursued by central or local government.   (Hoggett, 1990, p. 9)

We need not, indeed *do* not, assume that ministers sat down and read their post-Fordist management texts, and then drafted *WfP*. On the contrary, the white paper was a rushed and somewhat incoherent product of a pressing political need to solve a political crisis. Nevertheless, aspects of the *WfP* arrangements reflect management ideas that were in good currency at the time.

But what would the role of the centre be in a post-Fordist NHS? Certainly not operational management. Nor the formulation of an all-encompassing plan. Instead the centre would be concerned with maintaining and, where necessary, revising the 'rules of the game'. The aim would be to keep both purchasers and producers on their toes, to keep the playing field level and visible to all the potential players. There might also be a need to set, or ensure that someone else set, some quality and access standards. These would be part of the rules of the game, a safeguard against the danger that the internal market would run solely according to price incentives. Such a bundle of responsibilities would be quite novel, so it is worth asking how far the actual structures created by *WfP* are suitable for such a task.

Having established three possible roles for the centre (traditional, 'command' and post-Fordist) we can now deploy our key concepts (power, culture and uncertainty) to explore the most likely future developments. We are not, of course, saying that the central organisations (the Policy Board and Executive) will have to conform precisely with one of these three. Two of them (the command model and the post-Fordist) are in any case ideal types. The third (the traditional) is no more than the assemblage of ideas and practices which accumulated during roughly the first thirty years of the NHS's existence. We have no need to analyse the traditional role any further here, having dealt with it at length in earlier work and earlier chapters (Haywood and Hunter, 1982; Harrison, 1988a; Harrison, Hunter and Pollitt, 1990).

The *command model* is, in our view, most unlikely to be realised in its fully developed form. It may, however, gain ground as a creeping alternative to the post-Fordist provider market, especially if the latter gets off to an accident-prone start. At least one simulation of the NHS market, using real NHS 'players', seemed to indicate that quality and equity objectives would frequently take second place to crude financial pressures and other short term influences (Liddell and Parston, 1990). One conclusion drawn was that the 'internal market will not function smoothly' if individual players are simply left to act in isolation. Another was that the 'RHA has overall responsibility for setting performance criteria and performance measures' (East Anglian Regional Health Authority, 1990, p. 25). Both point to a measure of hierarchical co-ordination and control.

However, attempts to move decisively towards a full command model would almost certainly provoke tremendous resistance, and for little tangible political gain. Such a move would collide with both deeply rooted cultural assumptions and strong centres of autonomous power. The cultural assumptions are that districts have a considerable measure of autonomy and that doctors, rather than politicians, should determine who gets treated, when, where and how. The power relationships are the much-documented independence of the medical profession, with its attendant ability to delay, divert and dissolve centrally-promulgated priorities. Thus when, in mid-1991, the Prime Minister launched his 'Citizens Charter' the centre insisted on guaranteed maximum waiting times for operations but his Secretary of State for Health explained that 'These guaranteed times must be negotiated at the district level because they have to be supported by clinicians locally' (Timmins and Jones, 1991, p. 5).

Nor would the political gains in any way be likely to compensate those at the centre for the battles which would ensue from attempting such a transformation. A full command model would entail the centre laying down exactly the kind of explicit operational priorities which ministers of all political persuasions have consistently fought shy of. During the first thirty years the centre produced few well-defined priorities. The high water mark was probably the 'Priorities' document of 1976 (DHSS, 1976). This represented the climax of the belief in synoptic planning which characterised the late 1960s and early 1970s but on the whole it failed to constrain traditional local autonomy. After that there was a gradual and unannounced retreat from specific, quantified targets. Subsequently, in what may be regarded as the proto-command period after the introduction of general management, the centre changed tack and produced so many 'priorities' and 'initiatives' that the whole business had become something of a weary joke among the managers we interviewed during our 1986–89 study. The Management Board promised a single, limited set of national priorities, but this never appeared in public. In mid-1991 no less a person than Sir Roy Griffiths opined that 'There was no attempt to establish objectives at the centre . . . ' (quoted in May, 1991).

The elusiveness of a compact, operationally-meaningful set of national priorities should not surprise us. There are at least two reasons (in addition to medical resistance) which would deter any rational minister from attempting to promulgate any such thing. The first of these is the huge uncertainties which are necessarily involved. The second is the equally unavoidable assumption of increased responsibility for a set of decisions which are always likely to prove unpopular and contentious.

The uncertainties are both narrowly medical and broadly social. Medically, we still do not know what the effectiveness is (still less the relative cost-effectiveness) of many medical procedures. As indicated in Chapter 1, medical power rests largely on medical *inputs*, not effectiveness in terms of *outcomes* (see also Harrison, *et al.*, 1990, ch. 5). An elegant statement of the uncertainties around outcomes was made two decades ago in a milestone lecture by Archibald Cochrane, and it has been repeated from time to time ever since (Cochrane, 1972; Holland, 1983, p. xiv; Tomlin, 1991a and b). More broadly, we are not even sure that medical care is the answer to the problem. If the improvement of the health status of the population is the aim then giving attention to social issues such as diet, housing, lifestyles, environmental pollution and safety in the workplace may be as or more effective than increasing the resources put into medical care. Yet we understand the interaction between these other variables even less well than we understand the specific effectiveness of many medical interventions. The individual's social class position seems an important intervening variable, but how does it all work?

> The unanswered questions are essentially ones of linkages between structure, position in structure, values and attitudes, health-related behaviour and health status.   (Illsley, 1980, p. 4)

Uncertainty, then, made and makes health care an unpromising candidate for a Fordist, command-type treatment. It is as though Henry Ford were trying to run a Dearborn plant from which hundreds of different models were produced, often to loose specifications, with poor cost data and, in many cases, little or no reliable information about the performance of the vehicles on the road.

Yet even if 'production' decisions could be made with greater confidence there would still be significant political reasons for not wanting to run the NHS from the centre. As several commentators have pointed out, the rationing decisions which are inevitable in a cash-limited service largely free at the point of demand have always been made in a highly dispersed and only partly visible way (Klein, 1989). They are made bit by bit, by individual doctors and particular health authorities. They are not generally seen as 'political' – certainly not party-political – and they only infrequently attract national media coverage. To centralise a larger share of these decisions might yield some 'rationality gains', and might help close various 'implementation gaps' between nationally-declared policies and what actually goes on in Hexham or Horsham. However, it would also increase the visibility of rationing. Rationing decisions are never likely to be popular, and under a more centralised system they would be much more clearly identified with ministers and top level managers. This is not a privilege to which ministers and managers usually aspire. Under the *WfP* provider market the visibility of rationing may also increase, but at least it will remain a dispersed, fragmentary process where the responsibility can be pushed onto local managers.

Our conclusion, then, is that the command model is not likely to become the dominant one. Neither, however, is it likely entirely to disappear. To some extent it is always in the wings, a manifestation of central political pressures for public accountability, Treasury impatience at the escalating costs of the service or Department of Health frustration at its inability to reduce waiting lists, solve the problem of the hours worked by junior hospital doctors or whatever. Looking ahead to the provider market, the Public Accounts Committee, far from seeking 'hands off', recommended that:

> the Management Executive should develop a far more penetrating form of external budget review . . . this might be applied to authorities on a selective basis. (Committee of Public Accounts, 1990, p. vii)

When there is a 'scandal' or a financial 'crisis' or some glaring failure of service, the pressures on ministers to intervene can be very great. One thinks of the first set of DHSS-promulgated manpower ceilings in the early 1980s or the centre's demands for very detailed data when it set up the ill-fated waiting list initiative in the late 1980s. But these may be regarded as only spasmodic efforts at command – they are not comprehensive and neither are they continuous.

We turn now, therefore, to the other main contender as replacement for the traditional model – a post-Fordist centre devoted to the orchestration of a provider market. Such a centre would have an arm's length relationship with purchasers and providers. Following ministerial decisions determining the programme total for public expenditure, and the share of that total which was to go to the NHS, the centre would (as previously) allocate that resource to RHAs. But thereafter it would be for the latter to carry forward the job of 'setting performance criteria, monitoring the performance of the Health Service and evaluating its effectiveness' (Department of Health *et al.*, 1989, p. 13). Questioned by the Parliamentary Select Committee for Social Services in mid-1990 the then Secretary of State for Health said that the centre would not be monitoring the success or otherwise of NHS trusts or budget-holding GP practices:

> There will certainly be no central statistical monitoring. The social services committee will have to get used, like everyone in the service, to the idea of delegating responsibility to the hands of local managers and patients.   (Kenneth Clarke, quoted in MacLachlan, 1990)

Taken literally, this was a novel and puzzling doctrine. How can a Parliamentary Select Committee, a non-executive body, delegate anything, other, perhaps, than to another Parliamentary organ? And what, precisely, is to be delegated to patients?

When, in July 1990, five hundred senior NHS managers met with members of the Policy Board and the Executive to discuss progress with the white paper reforms similar 'arms-length' attitudes were struck. The Chief Executive chose an issue of high political salience – waiting lists – but made it clear whose task he thought it was to deal with the problem. Citing the then waiting list figures he said:

> This is simply not acceptable and the Management Executive's task for managers is to reduce waiting times. The contractual process can drive it down: you can specify clearly a maximum waiting time in the contracts.   (quoted in Millar, 1990a)

This kind of statement represents a fascinating blend of 50% post-Fordist management and 50% command. The centre is not going to tell managers exactly how to do it – it is simply indicating that they should use the contracts and get on with it. On the other hand the centre is certainly not allowing managers simply to respond to the dictates of the internal market, whatever they may be. On the contrary, it is saying, in effect, 'waiting lists are the thing – give them top priority' (see also O'Sullivan, 1991).

Of course, allocating money once a year will not be the only function for the centre. The Secretary of State has retained, for example, extensive patronage powers. These include the appointment of the chairs of trusts, the chairs and non-executive members of RHAs, and the chairs of DHAs. In the first round of appointments of regional non-executive members the Secretary of State favoured two groups, first, previous RHA members and, second, business managers (Millar, 1990b). These appointments unsurprisingly confirmed the Conservative Government's perception that what the running of the NHS still needed was the injection of more business acumen.

There is also the issue of pay. The Thatcherite government of the late 80s was keen to promote local pay flexibility. It openly declared its impatience with the Whitley system of national agreements (Millar, 1990c). Some increase in local flexibility may well be achieved, but that is a far cry from saying that central government will be able to relax its public expenditure interests in how one of the largest groups of workers in the country are paid. Even under a non-Thatcher Conservative administration the centre will surely continue to have a role here, though perhaps a marginally less prominent one than in the recent past.

However, the most interesting aspects of the post-*WfP* centre's role are probably those to do with the design and adjustment of the provider market. One can envisage a number of specific elements within this, for example:

(a) Issuing guidelines and regulations governing the contracting process.
(b) Adjudicating any particularly difficult or consequential disputes between parties to a contract.
(c) Ensuring that national minimum quality standards are developed and promulgated.
(d) Evaluating the introduction of major new technologies/services to the system, especially where the resource characteristics of these make them 'naturals' for super-regional specialty status.
(e) Co-ordinating any national campaigns or initiatives which may be adjudged necessary, e.g. screening programmes or educational campaigns on diet or sexually transmitted diseases.

Taken together these do indeed represent a considerably altered role for the centre. One might suppose that the first three of these tasks would decline over time. As managers gained experience in operating the market, and as a set of precedents and models were accumulated the amount of steering and fine-tuning required from the centre should diminish. But what are the chances that this vision will actually be realised? This question resolves itself into two parts: first, can the centre acquire the capacity to discharge these new tasks and, second, can it resist the pressures and temptations to intervene in other, additional ways? Our key concepts of power and culture again help us to assess the probabilities.

First, it is clear that the centre is almost as untrained and inexpert in the running of a provider market as is the rest of the NHS. This is, quite simply, because no such market has ever existed before, either in the UK or elsewhere, even on a pilot basis. The addition of the ubiquitous business people at every level from Policy Board to DHA may help somewhat – especially with the niceties of contracting – but the NHS 'market' will be a most unusual and distinctive one, to which lessons drawn from a business background may not apply in any straightforward way. So it is quite likely that all sorts of problems will crop up. The culture of the NHS has hitherto been that problems are commonly resolved by making regulations or guidelines which are developed in a fairly bureaucratic way and are then applied to the Service as a whole. It is an open question how far the Management Executive will be able to put this practice behind it, and how far managers at lower levels can wean themselves away from the habit of clearing things 'up the line'. Evidence from research into the post-1983 management reforms (Chapters 3 and 4) seems to indicate that for very local issues substantial devolution was possible, but that once an issue crossed a district boundary or involved a major capital scheme then 'referring up' remained as pervasive as ever. If this cultural predisposition continues then both the Management Executive and the RHAs may find themselves drawn into a morass of detailed adjudications and rule-makings.

The power relationships involved could easily reinforce this cultural tendency. There is little sign that the general public are willing to go along with the 'de-politicisation' of the NHS. It remains a central topic in the struggle between Conservative and Labour. Indeed, as of April 1992 Labour is making considerable political mileage out of the accusation that the Conservative Government is attempting to subvert the NHS into a 'commercial business' (Cook, 1990, p. 4). In this situation the pressure on the Policy Board to 'do something' or at least 'say something' when one aspect or another of the NHS receives adverse media attention will continue to be great. The 1990 ambulance strike illustrated this very clearly. At the beginning the then Secretary of State said it was a management matter, and tried to persuade the media to address their questions to the Chief Executive, Duncan Nichol. This stance collapsed almost immediately, and the political level was drawn in further and further, and more and more visibly. The Secretary of State was also quickly drawn in to the public controversy over fund-holding GPs 'queue-jumping' their patients in the new provider market (O'Sullivan, 1991).

It is just possible to imagine a situation where the internal market has settled in, the dividing line between the NHS and private health care is much more blurred by 'partnership' and other arrangements than it has been in the past, and information systems for both costs and achieved quality are far more advanced than at present. Perhaps the public could then learn not so readily to look to central government to remedy perceived deficiencies in the health care system. The probability of this scenario, however, seems low. In every developed western economy health care arrangements continue to be a matter of intense political interest and concern. And in the specific case of the NHS, starting down the path from 'here' to 'there' has already raised rather than dampened the temperature of the political environment. A more probable outcome than a truly post-Fordist centre is the continuance of something closer to the 1980s practice in which the centre:

(a)   still claims a strategic, objective-setting role but
(b)   in practice avoids the dangerous and difficult business of actually setting a limited set of prioritised objectives, progress towards which is measurable.
(c)   continues to give rhetorical support for decentralised, local management but
(d)   nevertheless intervenes fairly often to attempt to deal with issues within the Service which have become politically contentious.

This is not to say that the near future will bring no changes at all. The actual substance of the issues dealt with by the centre may alter considerably. The regulation of contracts and trusts will very likely become major concerns. But at a deeper level of analysis these issues may be seen as the new forms in which more traditional relationships and tensions are played out. The balance between what Klein, writing of the birth of the NHS, called 'bureaucratic control at the centre and freedom at the periphery to respond to local demands' may well move somewhat in favour of the latter (Klein, 1989, p. 12). But a revolutionary shift to 'hands off' post-Fordism remains improbable. Both cultural inertia and political rationality stand in the way, and each is reinforced by the uncertainties surrounding the delivery of an extraordinarily complex and sophisticated set of services.

RESOURCE MANAGEMENT

In earlier chapters we have discussed the sometimes painfully slow progress which has been made in persuading hospital doctors to play a more active and formally responsible role in managing the resources which, by their clinical decisions, they effectively commit. Our conclusions on this score have recently been largely confirmed by a evaluative study of the six resource management (RM) pilot sites carried out by a team from Brunel University. They acknowledged that, 'With hindsight the original initiative was grossly optimistic both about the timescales and the costs of RM' (Packwood *et al.*, 1991, p. 154).

In this chapter, however, we are looking to the future, and so the question about RM becomes one of its role within the post-*WfP* NHS. Officially RM has become even more important. *WfP* signalled a 'roll-out' of RM, with more than 130 major units being formally involved by early 1992 and others pursuing 'home grown' schemes of a similar character. RM was one of the few elements in *WfP* that actually received support from the Labour opposition (Cook, 1990, p. 18). Furthermore the wariness displayed by the medical profession over the notion of doctor-managers appears to have diminished. Among consultants directly involved with RM schemes there is evidently still caution about the demands on their time that participation makes, but despite agnosticism about the net benefits to patient care thus far, they remain optimistic about the future (Packwood *et al.*, 1991, p. 159). At the centre the bullishness of *WfP* has perhaps been shaded somewhat, but there is still an insistence on a rosy future. Giving evidence to the Public Accounts Committee during 1990 the NHS Chief Executive referred to a 'long evolutionary period' for RM but nevertheless foresaw a 'transformation' after 1993 (Committee of Public Accounts, 1990, p. 2). We would merely observe that 'after 1993' the RM initiative will be eight years old – a long period indeed.

How, if at all, does RM fit in with our three organisational models, the traditional, the Fordist and the post-Fordist? It actually accommodates itself quite well within the post-Fordist mould. Compared with the traditional way of running a hospital RM represents:

Two transformations: from an organisation based on a division of labour to one based on a division of knowledge; and from top-down to distributed control.   (Packwood *et al.*, 1991, p. 164)

The sub-unit becomes the hub of the organisation and collaboration and sharing of information between sub-units assumes the status of a key issue.

This is the vision, but not yet (on any widespread basis) the reality. Until now service priorities, in so far as they have been consciously planned at all, have been determined from the top down. Unless this habit can be broken the RM game may not seem worth playing, because the room for manoeuvre left for sub units may be so small (Packwood *et al.*, 1991, p. 168). In the post *WfP* NHS this game is likely to be played out across the purchaser/provider line. For it is the DHAs, as purchasing authorities, who are supposed to determine priorities. There is perhaps the beginnings of a paradox here – RM (or something like it) is essential for providers if they are to be able to cost their operations in detail and persuade multi-professional teams to 'own' the cost and quality targets that will be built into contracts. Yet the more purchasers are able over time to develop advanced contracting skills and exploit competition among providers the more tight may become the requirements the latter are obliged to meet – thus somewhat undermining the freedoms which RM currently proffers to clinical directorates and other sub-units.

However, this is still very speculative. The post-Fordist vision of a myriad of sophisticated contractual arrangements – some of a highly specialist 'short batch' type (Johnston and Lawrence, 1988) – has yet to be realised. In the beginning the provider market has been characterised by large block contracts with highly aggregated forms of pricing. In theoretical terms such contracts are often 'incomplete' in that they do not specify in detail the actions consequent on all future possible states of the world (Bartlett, 1991, p. 4). This in turn makes possible opportunistic behaviour by contractual parties who may be able to manipulate uncertainties to their advantage by selective or distorted disclosure of information. Bartlett argues that this is likely to favour providers over purchasers:

> Much of the information concerning quality of treatment is unobservable to outside scrutiny, and is the private and hidden information of the provider. The provider can take advantage of the hidden nature of this information, and raise the average cost of delivering services within the block contract above that which would be attained if information about levels of quality were easily observable.   (Bartlett, 1991, p. 17)

Furthermore the making and re-making of large block contracts are matters so consequential for the organisations concerned that highly centralised, oligopolistic negotiations are the order of the day. Top management on both purchaser and provider sides are anxious to keep the other side in business; indeed from mid 1990 the Government began to urge managers to behave conservatively and not to depart radically from previous referral patterns (purchaser behaviour will be further discussed below). For the present, therefore, it could be said that the NHS 'market' is still heavily flavoured with bureaucracy and hierarchy. Even after a general election victory in April 1992 giving the Conservatives a comfortable, if reduced, majority it is likely that the NHS market will develop incrementally and that 'steady state' will not be overturned completely in the first few years of the reforms.

GENERAL MANAGERS' AGENDAS

The one observation about managers in the post-*WfP* environment for which there is already abundant empirical evidence is that they are grossly overloaded. In the period since the January 1989 publication, the government has been obliged to make several retreats from the absurdly optimistic timetables it set out at that time. Senior managers are having to deal not only with contracts, RM, consultant job descriptions, quality assurance, new financing formulae, and re-constituted health authorities but also with yet another round of reorganisation. The last-named arises from at least three sources. In the first place there are the numerous internal reorganisations deemed necessary in order to shape up for the new market environment (e.g. where and how are contracts going to be handled within the organisation?). Second, principally but not exclusively at regional level, there are the changes consequent upon the new subordination of FHSAs to RHAs. Last, but not least, anticipation of the market led to something of a 'merger fever'. District mergers or inter-district consortia have been one way of forming larger, more powerful purchasing entities. On the provider side a tremendous amount of managerial time has gone into consideration of what, if anything, should go forward in the way of trust applications. These processes have frequently been fairly conflictual, with substantial portions of the local consultant body coming out in public against the management line (e.g. O'Sullivan, 1990).

All in all we suggest there is good reason to suppose that for many managers some of the features of the period 1983–88 will recur. Once more there is clearly an initial period in which reorganisation itself is a very time-consuming task. Alongside that, finance will surely remain at the top of most agendas, and, indeed, become (if that is possible) an even more intense preoccupation. A key feature of the market is that the global budget is fixed by government in advance. Hospitals will thus be competing to reduce cost and increase output but without any prospect of their efforts increasing the total size of the cake. By the middle of 1991 there were familiar signs of DHAs running out of cash (Brown, 1991). What is more, purchasers and providers will probably continue to be desperately short of qualified finance and IT staff (Committee of Public Accounts, 1990).

Attention to finance is therefore likely to become even more obsessive than that which we found in 1986–88. At that time a number of general managers and others indicated that this state of affairs inevitably reduced the amount of time and attention which managers could give to issues of quality. We foresee this happening again. In many ways the kind of market that has been set up encourages a new kind of complicity between managers and doctors over quality. Of course, managers could use their access to medical audit and other clinical information to make a big issue out of quality. But is it not more likely that, with the other calls on their attention, managers will be more than content to go for the outward form – a medical audit committee with minutes and broad-brush reports – and leave what actually goes on within this shell largely to doctors? Equally, is this not exactly what would suit many doctors? Why should either side get into deep and sensitive waters when there are so many other issues demanding urgent attention? It is interesting to note that patient outcomes 'are not yet a routine part of RM data collection, and that if they are to become so special exercises will be required' (Packwood *et al.*, 1991, p. 137). Nor can purchasers be relied on to break this complicity. They, too, are going to be primarily concerned with money. Of course, they will also want reassurance about clinical quality, but our speculation is that in many cases it will be quite rational for purchasers to look for an essentially formal pledge of minimum quality rather than more aggressively seeking detailed comparative quality information with a view to pushing all its providers towards optimal quality levels.

A further feature of general managers' agendas during the late 1980s was the extent to which they were determined not so much by the particulars of local problems as by the need to respond to the stream of 'initiatives' coming down from the centre. A crucial question for managers' agendas during the 1990s is the extent to which the centre is willing and able to refrain from this kind of behaviour. This was discussed at length in the section on hierarchy. It is impossible to make a confident prediction here, but our suspicion is that the political temptations to intervene will, in the early years of a controversial reform, prove very hard to resist. The post-Fordist, 'hands-off' rhetoric is currently fashionable but it remains to be seen whether the centre's actual behaviour will follow. As suggested earlier, *WfP* is an awkward mixture of the command and post-Fordist models. General managers may well be left with the job of trying to reconcile these inconsistencies whilst simultaneously overseeing the day-to-day running of an exceedingly complex set of services. It is not an enviable task.

PUBLIC ACCOUNTABILITY AND THE ROLE OF HEALTH AUTHORITIES

The one thing that most students of the NHS learned by reading the research literature of the 1980s was that health authority members were seldom powerful and only intermittently influential. The real power at the periphery lay not with the appointed members but with varying combinations of doctors and managers (Harrison, 1988a; Harrison, Hunter and Pollitt, 1990). In a sense, therefore, the disinterested observer might say 'so what?' to the changes in health authority membership announced in *WfP*. We would have some sympathy with this assessment, but would wish to qualify it by setting the issue within a broader frame. Thus we would not attempt to argue that members were now likely suddenly to become dominantly powerful but rather would observe that the ꞁꞁꞁꞁꞁꞁꞁꞁꞁꞁ ꞁꞁ ꞁꞁꞁꞁꞁ ꞁꞁꞁꞁꞁꞁꞁꞁꞁꞁ ꞁꞁ but the latest manifestation of the older and larger problem of democratic representation within the NHS.

The early history of this problem is now reasonably well known. During the original design of the Service, Herbert Morrison favoured a major role for democratically elected local authorities. But this strand of Labour thought was defeated by two arguments and one pressure group. The arguments, deployed by the then Minister for Health, Aneurin Bevan, were, first, that a centrally controlled NHS would be more efficient and, second that it would also be better placed to provide a uniform set of services throughout the country. The pressure group was the medical profession, which left ministers in no doubt that it was not prepared to serve under the direction of local councillors (Klein, 1989; Pater, 1981).

Despite occasional subsequent interest in 'democratising' the NHS (mainly from the Labour or Liberal parties, or from individual academics) the democratic component remained vestigial. By the time of *WfP* each DHA contained four to six local authority members (part-time and unpaid) but they were nominated by the councils concerned rather than being directly elected. Following *WfP* three important changes occurred. First, members were no longer appointed because they were councillors or trade unionists – they were all chosen to be members in a personal capacity, so local authority nomination ceased. Second, DHA and general managers themselves became members of the authority. Third, the total number of non executives per authority was reduced from around 16 to five. The new DHAs were to have a lean, managerial appearance.

The authors of *WfP* evidently considered that relevant skills for members included the kinds of financial management and contracting skills most often acquired in private sector business. Implicitly they valued knowledge of the local political system less highly. Obviously alternative views are possible – and the transition from Thatcher to Major may have marginally reduced the emphasis on 'businessmen'. However, rather than argue the merits of this here it may be more useful to follow the *WfP* logic to the next stage. That is, can individuals with those skills be persuaded to serve? Early evidence is that a reasonable number can – a fifth or more of early non-executive appointments, at both district and regional levels, were from business backgrounds (Millar, 1990a) – and this figure excludes any business men or women who were already members of the preceding health authorities and were reappointed. Whether they stay is another matter, and whether their skills enable them to shape policy and practice another again.

On this last point we would express some doubt. The main reasons why rank and file members lacked clout are undiminished (Ham, 1985, pp. 157–160; Hunter, 1984a, pp. 41–67). They are not particularly special to the health service, but may be present there to an even greater degree than in some other public services (Day and Klein, 1987). The non-executives will still be part-timers dealing with full time managers and doctors. The difficulties of mastering the complexities of running a health authority, perhaps particularly in so far as decisions trespass onto what have hitherto been medical domains, remain. The general manager can speak on behalf of the staff. The finance director can speak for financial probity and necessity. Doctors can rest on the authoritative judgements of their profession. Prior to *WfP* local councillors could at least claim some sort of political legitimacy, however indirect. But what legitimacy can a non-executive business member claim? Their accounting or contracting skills are soon likely to be at least matched by the full time officers reporting to the general manager and/or the finance director. Beyond that they would seem to have no constituency and no other distinctive resource, and therefore little power. The notion that possession of specialist skills alone will give them much leverage in an organisation which bristles with all manner of special professional skills appears over-optimistic.

It may well be that the role and composition of DHAs was one of the less thought-through elements of the white paper. After all, relegation to Chapter 8 of *WfP* could be interpreted as an indication that trusts, contracts and the rest were the main focus of the government's attention, and changes at authority level a minor consequential. If so, the developing public debate following *WfP*, together with the ideological shift from Thatcher to Major, compelled some re-thinking. Gradually the importance of DHAs as 'champions of the people' (as Kenneth Clarke put it) gained recognition in government pronouncements, and the rapt attention accorded to the details of provider competition began to be complemented by a concern for the role of the DHA as purchaser for the community.

Early surveys of DHA members uncovered some interesting features of the initial days of the new authorities. Asked by a Warwick University team about their knowledge gaps members put public health and contracting at the top of their lists (*Health Service Journal*, 1991). Meanwhile King's Fund research seemed to indicate that in some districts non-executive members still had strong interests on the provider side, and that this might be complicating the development of a distinctive purchaser emphasis (Ham, 1991 a and b).

In sum, it would appear that the new-style DHA, devoted to the purchaser role and the promotion of public health, has got off to rather a late start. It was not the main focus of the original political interest in *WfP*. It is being inserted into a Service which has suffered from acute provider dominance since birth. It is handicapped by informational, methodological and conceptual backwardness: 'Well into the first year of contracting, there is no consensus on the best methods of assessing needs or measuring outcomes' (Tomlin, 1991a). Last, but not least, the new DHA is supposed to champion the people's needs but lacks any representative element that might legitimise its role in speaking for those needs. On the contrary, DHAs are in some danger of being merely 'ivory tower contracting bodies governed by a small group of managers and non-executive members, many of whom have come into the NHS from business backgrounds' (Ham, 1991b, p. 16).

Late in 1990 the Labour opposition produced its own proposals for running the NHS. These were updated in an alternative white paper, *Your Good Health*, published in February 1992. Labour's proposals gave DHAs a prominent role in implementing, in partnership with local authorities, a wide range of preventative and health-promoting measures. Representatives of local authorities would be restored to DHAs which would become 'more broadly-based public authorities' (Cook, 1990, p. 21). In the longer term some of the functions of RHAs might be devolved to Labour's new elected regional assemblies.

Whilst this alternative Labour future certainly gives more explicit attention to the nature of the public accountability of health authorities than did *WfP* it still gives rise to some of the concerns identified in the preceeding paragraphs. Nothing is said to indicate any change in the actual process of DHA decision making, so a skeptical view might be that the change in membership was little more than the swap of one not very powerful group of people for another.

The proposal for devolution of functions to an elected regional assembly raises many questions. Which functions? What would the relationship be between the regional assemblies and the centre? It also re-addresses a fundamental aspect of the original 1948 settlement in a novel way. The representative bodies of the medical profession were always mistrustful of local political control, though they accepted the kind of rather distant, national political control which Bevan proposed. But under the 1990 *Fresh Start* document (Cook, 1990) it would be regional, not local supervision, and it would follow more than 40 years of relatively benign experience of a politically structured and funded national service. No doubt there would still be medical resistance to the idea, and ritual protestations of the need to 'keep politics out of health care'. Yet there seems no reason why a determined and secure government could not insist that such a reform should go through. Once implemented there would, for the first time, be a force within the NHS which could offer a source of legitimate authority alternative to that of the medical profession. It is impossible to forecast what the outcome of such an innovation would be, but the new interface between political authority and medical authority would surely be at least as lively as that between medicine and management was during the 1980s. An elected element within the body of the NHS itself would constitute both a change in the balance of power and, probably, the beginnings of a significant cultural shift.

In sum, many details of the Labour alternative remained unclear up to the general election in April 1992. We can say with confidence that had a Labour government been elected managers would have continued to have a prominent role, but we could not be sure of the instruments they would have at their disposal, nor how a novel, democratic element would be fitted in. Such considerations are academic in the face of Labour's electoral defeat at the general election. The Party is likely to review fundamentally its policy on the NHS since by 1997 the NHS reforms will have become embedded. Hints to this effect have already been given by the Party's shadow health secretary, Robin Cook (Cook, 1992).

'CONSUMERS' AND THE NEW MANAGEMENT ARRANGEMENTS

Since the late 1980s Conservative ministers have laid great rhetorical emphasis on 'consumer choice' in the public service sector. In mid-1991 this culminated in John Major's announcement of a 'Citizen's Charter' aimed at raising standards right across the public services (Timmins, 1991). Previously, of course, the NHS reforms had themselves been presented under the banner *Working for Patients*, and as indicated in earlier chapters, the consumerist thread can be traced back at least as far back as the Griffiths Report of 1983.

As many commentators have pointed out, Conservative consumerism has tended to be of a very particular and somewhat limited type (e.g. Pollitt, 1988). It has not, for example, had much truck with the idea of extending the legal rights of public service consumers. Nor has it exhibited enthusiasm for public subventions to representative consumer organisations. Consumer *participation* in what the government defines as management issues has certainly been frowned upon – managers must be free to manage. Conservative consumerism has been found focussed mainly on providing the individual public service user with more information about services and more 'choice', where choice is conceived largely in terms of the opportunity of 'exit', especially exit to private sector alternatives.

Thus, despite the consumerist rhetoric around *WfP* no new legal rights for NHS patients have been created, and neither have any new organisational arrangements been made to strengthen their collective voice in the affairs of either purchasing DHAs or providing units. Community Health Councils – survivors of the 1974 reorganisation – have pressed to be given a formally recognised and entrenched role in monitoring the quality of services, but the government has resisted:

> the Department has always indicated that, given the sensitivities of the medical profession on the establishment of medical audit committees, there was no immediate prospect of CHCs – or indeed any lay person – being involved in the process. (personal communication from Association of Community Health Councils for England and Wales, 4 April, 1990)

Of course, not all is gloomy on the consumer front. In a number of places local management has moved to include the consumer voice in decision-making by RHAs or DHAs. Oxford and South West Thames regions are involving CHCs in the drafting of service specifications. Some districts are seeking CHC comments as an input to the contracting process. Many provider units have carried out or are carrying out consumer surveys of one type or another.

Yet virtually all these developments are at the discretion of management – where management decides to exclude or ignore the local CHC there is little the latter can do effectively to contest the issue. At the time of writing CHCs are bridling at an apparent trend for DHAs to make greater use of private meetings from which press and public are excluded (Ham, 1991a, p. 23). The frustrations of this position were clearly expressed at the 1991 annual conference of the Association of Community Health Councils in England and Wales (ACHCEW), where the visiting junior health minister got a hostile reception (Tomlin, 1991b). True to the Conservative model outlined above, the minister declared that the ACHCEW had no right to expect government funding. He also rejected a conference resolution seeking a statutory right for CHCs to participate in the debate at DHA meetings (Labour had already promised to restore the CHCs observer status for the whole of DHA meetings).

In sum, the new NHS provider market does not as yet offer CHCs any firm foothold in the crucial processes of standard setting and contract formulation. Some local managements are taking CHCs into their confidence, but there is no guarantee that this will become the norm. In this respect CHCs may make a public fuss (first dimension of power) but are unlikely to be able to secure their interests if and when management resists. On the second and third dimensions their power appears negligible. In cultural terms it seems probable, taking the arguments in this section and the previous one together, that the NHS will continue to operate a Fordist, provider-dominated mode of service delivery for a good while yet. Consumer views may well be collected much more assiduously than in the past, but mainly in the managerially-malleable form of the survey questionnaire. Notions of direct consumer representation (and still more participation) have no real place in the new provider market.

MANAGEMENT AND THE MEDICAL PROFESSION

The analysis of changing power relations within healthcare organisations is often conducted on the basis of a search for signs of what is being taken away from doctors (Alford, 1975 was an early and well-known example; parts of our own works also follow this line, for instance Harrison, 1988a). If, however, the most is to be made of this kind of approach it is vital that the elements of 'doctor power' are separated out and examined one by one. Thus, in terms of Chapters 1 and 5, we need to monitor both the scope and the domain of the profession's power, at both macro- and micro-levels.

Previous chapters have identified and distinguished between some of these different elements. At a macro-level the medical profession operates as a highly persuasive and powerful pressure group. It is powerful because it can threaten to withdraw co-operation from government in activities where its monopoly expertise is irreplaceable, at least in the short term. Its power and persuasiveness are both fuelled by its expertise, its resources (because it is a rich pressure group) and by its cultural status (which means that it is usually perceived by the public as a responsible professional body rather than, say, a grasping, self-interested trade union).

However, at this macro-level the medical profession is still, ultimately, just another pressure group. It is frequently not even a united one: from the very beginnings of the NHS ministers have sometimes been able to drive wedges between the BMA and the Royal Colleges or GPs and hospital doctors. What is more, the medical bodies in London (just like other trade unions) cannot always 'deliver' or discipline their membership (a point we will return to in a moment). Thus at the national level the profession can be, and on occasion has been, decisively defeated. General management was introduced against its express wishes, and the provider market is an even more vivid example of central government's ability to introduce major changes to which the profession is vigorously, at times almost hysterically, opposed. The introduction, in 1985, of limitations on the drugs that doctors could prescribe under the NHS is a third example of 'defeat' at national level.

Whilst there has been no dramatic collapse in the power of the profession's peak associations it seems likely that for some years there has been a gradual decline. This stems from a number of factors. In the deep background there may be, as Chapter 5 suggests, a weakening in the cultural authority of doctors. Ideological shifts have brought into question both the effectiveness of medical expertise and the accuracy of the doctors' claim that medical interests are automatically at one with those of the wider community. The then Secretary of State for Health felt emboldened to play on this theme in the immediate aftermath of *WfP*, when he accused the BMA, in particular, of always being opposed to progressive change. In addition, the medical bodies have found themselves lobbying from within an increasingly crowded policy space. The NHS is a multi-professional organisation and the nurses and other clinical and technical professions have continuously developed their own lobbying strength. The medical profession remains the best-heeled, most entrenched group but it no longer enjoys the degree of domain overlordship it did 30 or more years ago. Furthermore, the relative extent of its domain may be waning. The hospital is the throne of the medical empire, but for more than 20 years now governments (and others) have emphasised the need to give priority to community-based forms of care. In the community sector, as some of the research projects cited earlier have demonstrated, medical dominance is not as marked as in the acute hospital. To date, however, this has been quite a slow shift in priorities, and public concern with the hospital sector has remained very strong – and exploitable by 'shroud-waving' doctors.

This last point brings us directly to consideration of medical influence at the micro-level. Arguably it is here, rather than at the macro-level, where doctors have proved themselves most powerful and resistant to policy change. The basic building blocks of this local power were set out in Chapter 1. With just a few carefully circumscribed exceptions only doctors may diagnose, admit, prescribe and discharge. Only doctors may admit new doctors to the profession. Only doctors can certify an institution fit for the purposes of medical training. Only a doctor may legitimately comment on the quality of another doctor's work. Taken together these 'onlys' – manifestations of the original, government-conferred monopoly – constitute a formidable power base. They create a whole network of dependencies and potential dependencies, which the profession has assiduously cultivated and protected. Thus they mean, for example, that the work patterns of many other occupational groups are extensively shaped or even directly controlled by the profession. If the consultant decides to admit a patient, if the surgeon decides to bring forward the date of the operation, if the physician prescribes such-and-such a drug regime, if the doctor refers the patient to the physiotherapist or the hospital dietician – all these decisions and many more cause work for others. They also commit resources, so that in aggregate, as was indicated in Chapter 2, 'policy' may become little more than the accumulation of thousands of 'medical' micro-decisions. Managers may try to persuade doctors to do more or less, to bear in mind the cost of this or that procedure, to consider the effects of their decisions on the overstretched nursing staff and so on, but when the chips are down managerial power to enforce such advice has always been very limited.

It is important to note that this micro-level power is not at all closely articulated with the power of the medical peak associations in London. The latter cannot turn it on or off, or direct the clinical decisions of the rank and file in any comprehensive or immediate way. Of course, extreme behaviour by individual practitioners can be disciplined, though the record shows that this is rare. For the majority of doctors the Royal Colleges can develop guidelines, protocols and so on, but despite considerable acceleration in this type of activity in recent years the coverage of such advice is still extremely patchy, and monitoring of compliance is the exception rather than the rule.

The impacts of this micro-level power have been visible throughout the processes and cases described in this book. The 'implementation gap' is much more a product of the profession's micro-freedoms than it is of its macro-lobbying power. As countless managers and nurses have said to us during our fieldwork, 'It's no use if you can't get the doctors to go along'. Medical micro-power is essentially conservative – it is a power to resist change that comes from outside, to resist not necessarily by battles at meetings and other 'first face' campaigns (though they may also occur) but rather by silent, individualistic non-compliance – a 'second face' refusal to become engaged or involved. That is one reason why it is so hard to beat – medical micro-power is not organised influence. There is no 'central brain' or committee to which reformers can address themselves. The situation is more like that depicted in Handy's ideal type of a 'person culture':

> The psychological contract states that the organisation is subordinate to the individual and depends on the individual for its existence. The individual can leave the organisation but the organisation seldom has the power to evict the individual. Influence is shared and the power-base, if needed, is usually expert; that is, individuals do what they are good at and are listened to on appropriate topics.   (Handy, 1976, p. 184)

Given this background the question we must now address is how the changes envisaged in *WfP* are likely to affect the macro- and micro-power of doctors, and, equally, how they will alter the roles played by managers. A preliminary answer would be that *WfP*, whatever else it may achieve, has clearly already further enhanced the prominence of management roles. Managers will and are already taking the lead in negotiating the contracts on which so much else will depend. Because services will be provided according to contract there is an unmistakable need to define and cost the work that is performed, including medical work, more precisely than ever before. In a general way, therefore, the work of doctors is bound to become more transparent to managers. RM is only one manifestation, albeit an important one, of this general tendency.

We should not be satisfied, however, with such a general answer. Though *WfP* may be a managers' charter in broad terms it is already clear that the tide of managerialism is likely to undermine some sections of the medical ramparts more than others. At a national, macro level, two points are worthy of particular note. First, as indicated above, the medical profession's frontal resistance to the *WfP* changes has not been successful. The DoH went ahead; the first batch of NHS trusts were approved in 1991, followed by a second wave in April 1992 and operational guidelines for designing contracts were circulated to health authorities and all manner of financial adjustments were made to approximate a 'level playing field' for the launch of the internal market. In sum, by April 1992 the new policies could be said to be largely in place.

Second, the Royal Colleges have taken on a particular role with respect to 'quality'. They have accepted a responsibility for developing quality controls in the new medical market place, and have accepted central government money to assist them perform this function (Tomlin, 1990; Pollitt, 1991). Briefly, health care quality assurance is to continue to be approached in two very different ways. Non-medical quality will be covered by a variety of schemes and techniques including Total Quality Management (TQM), voluntary accreditation (where the King's Fund has set up a scheme) and a range of 'consumerist' initiatives (NHS Management Executive, 1989). Medical quality, however, will apparently remain apart. 'The quality of medical work can only be reviewed by a doctor's peers' (Department of Health, 1989). And the Royal Colleges will lay down appropriate general guidelines, standards and protocols (e.g. Royal College of Physicians, 1989; Royal College of Surgeons, 1989).

Quality is an important issue in several ways. It is important to users of the NHS because the prospect of an internal market driven by price alone, without any reliable measures of quality, is a frightening one. But quality is also a crucial issue at the doctor/manager interface. In the past, medical or clinical quality was definitely part of the profession's sacred ground. In medicine, as in several other professions, managers were not allowed into the temple. Now, in medicine and elsewhere, the boundary is beginning to be crossed (Pollitt, 1990b). For while the first impression from *WfP* is that medical audit will be for doctors only a closer reading shows that this is unlikely to be wholly true in practice (Pollitt, 1991).

To begin with, it ought to be remembered that audit is being introduced throughout the NHS not because of some sudden upsurge of interest in it on the part of rank and file doctors. It is being introduced because *WfP* says that every district shall have a medical audit committee. The implications of the government's pressure are different at national and local levels.

At national level the government's insistence that every district should practice what had formerly been a voluntary, minority pursuit within the profession put the Royal Colleges in an awkward position. It would not look good to take a stance of outright opposition to government's demands for greater attention to quality. There was a reasoned fear that the new market pressures *would* lead to a fall in standards, and responsible medical leaders could see the need to guard against that. Some of them were also convinced of the need for more audit anyway – for the profession to shepherd its strays more carefully. Tactically, there was also a distinct danger that government would respond with some form of *external* quality review – perhaps an inspectorate or a beefed-up Health Advisory Service – and that this mechanism would be directly controlled by the DoH. Would it not be better to take the government's money and keep the whole sensitive business within the established medical network? In taking this line, however, the Colleges were also running the risk of at least mild incorporation. They were doing the government's bidding and taking money for it. It was noticeable, throughout the wrangling that followed publication of *WfP*, that medical audit was just about the only part of the package on which the DoH and the national medical bodies were in broad agreement. But would the Colleges be able to carry the rank and file with them? Their main weapon was accreditation for training. If a unit did not satisfy the relevant college in respect of its arrangements for medical audit, then training status might be refused. But how far would the Colleges insist on the substance (e.g. evidence that specific methods were being used, or specified standards were being attained) and how far would they rest content with the outward form (existence of an audit committee that kept regular minutes etc)? These are delicate questions of intra-professional relationships which cannot yet be answered.

At the local level the quality issue will make a more direct impact on the manager/doctor interface. Managers will have to satisfy themselves (as part of contract negotiations if nothing else) that medical quality assurance procedures are in place and working; managers, and probably health authority members, will want access to at least the aggregate data which emerges from the audit process. There are also important implications in the new DHA role as the 'people's purchaser'. Early indications are that this will legitimate quite large-scale intrusions by DGMs into territory formerly claimed by public health doctors. Managers will now need to play an active part in the process of assessing community needs.

Finally, there is the question of monitoring the provision of contractually agreed services. 'Management should be able to initiate an independent professional audit, for example where there is cause to question the quality or cost-effectiveness of a service' (Department of Health *et al.*, 1989, p. 41). As audit progresses aggregate data will be used as part of the process of costing treatment plans for a given population. At this stage, as an experienced consultant and audit project officer put it:

> For this to work purchasers must insist on nationally agreed minimum standards or unrestricted access to the information to derive quality measures from each provider unit. (Frater and Spiby, 1990, p. 1684)

Furthermore, districts may be asked to open themselves to investigation by the Audit Commission, either as part of a national study of a chosen issue, or as a local audit. Audit Commission studies may well include 'medical' topics (their first was on day surgery) and be supported by expert medical advisors (Smith, 1990).

Taken together these developments constitute a significant incursion into the medical domain. They represent a trimming of doctors' micro-power, because they open a management window, albeit an aggregated and anonymised one, onto those core medical activities of diagnosis, admissions, prescribing therapies and deciding on discharges. The dependence of managers (and, ultimately, the public) on doctors for authoritative reassurance on the quality of medical practice will henceforth be less absolute than in the past. Locally doctors will be obliged to yield at least some systematic information to management, and at national level the Royal Colleges have been persuaded by central government to play an important part in promulgating the whole process.

Nor is quality the only issue where doctors' micro-power is under challenge. The freedoms of the 'person culture' are to be constrained in other ways. Merit or distinction awards are currently made to more than a third of consultants. They are made on grounds of clinical excellence, and the highest of the four levels of award (C, B, A and A+) can add as much as 95% (A+) to the basic salary (C = 18%; B = 40%; A = 70%). Since 1948 merit awards have been made on the basis of judgements by a professional committee. The criteria by which these judgements have been made have never been precisely stated. In other words substantial additions to consultant salaries have been decided upon entirely within the profession, according to its own, essentially 'private' criteria.

WfP announced the opening of negotiations with the profession to change the way this system worked. The government proposed, *inter alia*, to add as a new criterion for the first, C-level award, 'a commitment to the management and development of the service' (Department of Health *et al.*, 1989, p. 44). It also intended to place managers on the regional and national committees which, respectively, nominate individuals for award and make the final decisions. Here, therefore, we see the injection of a managerial component into the profession's own system of advancement. This could be seen as a move on two levels. On the first, and most obvious, it extends the scope of managers' power – now they are to have a regular say in the nomination of consultants for C awards. Second, it represents one piece of a jigsaw of actions intended, eventually, to change the individualist culture of the medical profession. For it will oblige all doctors who want to 'get on' to give some thought and effort to management as well as to purely clinical matters. The once common belief among doctors that management is 'other' (and is there purely to facilitate clinicians rather than having any priorities of its own) should be further undermined and reduced.

Finally, there is the issue of job descriptions. The standard consultant contract of employment has hitherto been extremely vague as to the duties to be performed.

This is exactly what would be predicted for a 'person culture'. It leaves individual doctors plenty of room to invent their own jobs and pursue their own particular interests. *WfP*, however, heralded a change:

> every consultant should have a fuller job description than is commonly the case at present. This will need to cover their responsibility for the quality of their work, their use of resources, the extent of the services they provide for NHS patients and the time they devote to the NHS.   (Department of Health *et al.*, 1989, p. 42)

It would certainly be an exaggeration to claim that these several changes mean that doctors are now pinned down and shorn of their former autonomy. Much of their defensive power at the micro-level remains. More often than not their specialist knowledge is still effectively irreplaceable. Nor are there any eager candidates – certainly not managers – for the heavy responsibilities and painful uncertainties necessarily involved in day-to-day individual clinical decision-making or the micro-rationing which inevitably accompanies it. Managers and politicians alike remain dependent on the medical profession in these important respects. But the scope of its autonomy does appear to be diminishing. This trend was already apparent before *WfP* (Harrison and Schulz, 1989) but the foregoing analysis makes it seem likely that *WfP* represents an acceleration in the process. As one manager said to us during fieldwork, 'we've got them surrounded now'. The relative importance of the medical domain may also be slightly reduced, partly because of the increased emphasis on community care but partly too because of another long term trend:

the physician alone can no longer cope with the new task domains. This is particularly true when we focus on the most complex of health organisations, the hospital. The history of the modern hospital is the history of the steady decline of the physician's hierarchic power to control his [sic] work environment.   (Freddi, 1989, p. 8)

Thus we see *WfP* as significantly different from the introduction of general management in the mid 1980s. As our research showed, Griffiths Mark One created general managers and an accompanying rhetoric of managerialism, but did not actually provide those managers with any major new instruments for engaging with the micro-power of the medical profession. *WfP*, by contrast, does begin to provide those instruments. The combination of contracts, management participation in the assessment of public needs, management access to medical audit, consultant job descriptions and the inclusion of managerial criteria in the discretionary award process probably will, at last, 'shift the frontier' between medical and management power (Harrison, 1988a). Nevertheless, as noted in Chapter 5, the ability of the medical profession to find new means of exerting its micro-power should not be underestimated.

Before leaving this topic it is necessary to refer again to the post-Fordist and command models. Why have they not featured in our discussion of the medical profession? The short answer is that they are both models of management, not of a profession. One of the problems of applying such business-derived models to the NHS is precisely that they have no place for the kind of autonomy which the medical profession has hitherto enjoyed. Thus they fit the 'upper levels' of the NHS much more comfortably than they do the grass roots of day-to-day health care activity. As indicated earlier, the post-Fordist model grows out of a task culture, while the command model derives from a bureaucratic culture. Both are 'foreign' to the local person-culture in which doctors have wielded their micro-level powers. Yet they are not, so to speak, equidistant from traditional medical beliefs. We would argue that the post-Fordist model is not as alien as is the command model. This is because the post-Fordist model does allow for considerable freedom at the periphery. Specialised units run by local networks of experts are very much part of a post-Fordist world. Questioned by the Public Accounts Committee at the end of 1989 the NHS Chief Executive was clearly sympathetic to this approach:

So some of the large [hospital] campuses, whilst enjoying the benefits of inter-relationships clinically, can be broken down into managerial components by division . . . in many ways the whole purpose of involving doctors in the resource management initiative is to pin down and gain the benefits of cohesiveness and smallness around the clinical function within a much larger configuration.   (Committee of Public Accounts, 1990, p. 19)

Within this model, then, how units organised themselves would not be a matter for central intervention, always assuming service price and quality were satisfactory. Here, to be optimistic, could be a basis for a new concordat between medical power and managerial power. But for it to work well RM, or something similar, would have to develop in a direction, and at a speed, that our earlier analysis suggests to be unlikely.

CONCLUDING REFLECTIONS

This has been a long chapter, so no more than a very brief summary is needed here. We have found some evidence of a diminution of medical macro-power. But this is neither a dramatic nor a sudden development, and leaves the professional medical lobby still strong, though not quite as daunting an opponent as it may once have appeared. Occasional milestones mark the trend – the introduction of general management, the imposition of the limited list for prescribing, the government's refusal to compromise in any major way on the *WfP* proposals, the imposition of a new contract on GPs.

At the local level the picture is more complicated, and we are conscious that our interpretation is fragile. In general, we see the defensive micro-power of the medical profession holding up quite well through to the end of the 1980s. It is true that the concept of clinical freedom had been marginally narrowed in one or two areas (Harrison and Schulz, 1989) but in their relations with local managers both consultants and GPs remained conspicuously autonomous. In hospital settings doctors were the one group of staff over whom general managers were not regularly able to exert their authority. Neither were hospital doctors much ensnared by performance indicators, management budgeting, annual reviews or any of the other 1980s attempts to strengthen the 'command' aspects of management.

WfP, however, appears to mark a genuine watershed. It puts several additional levers of power and persuasion into managers' hands, in a way which Griffiths Mark 1 did not. These are not overwhelming powers, and we predict no spectacular collapse of the medical citadel. Even if used with skill and determination it would probably take some years before a general manager could hope to exert a regular, systematic and substantial influence on clinical workloads, clinical quality or clinical priorities. In many cases we imagine individual general managers will lack either the skill or the determination – most likely the latter, in the light of the rest of their overloaded agendas. Nevertheless, for the first time the basis for trimming the variance of local medical practice is there, and no doubt some will try to use it.

Meanwhile the fortunes of managers as a group have certainly waxed considerably over the last decade. The 'diplomat' model of the administrator (which emerged from the studies of the 70s and early '80s – Harrison, 1988a) is now almost dead. Quite what it has been replaced with may not yet be clear, but the status, powers (and, of course *pay*) of senior NHS managers have unmistakably grown. The introduction of general management was a crucial step in increasing the authority of managers over nurses and other professional groups, except for the doctors. Managers have successfully laid claim to a whole series of activities as 'management issues', so that there is now a distinct sphere of management action and authority in a way that, even 15 years ago, there was not.

What, though, of the medical citadel? If our above analysis is correct then the 1990s may see a gradual but significant shift of the medico-management frontier in favour of managers. Even to move, say, halfway towards the position in which the frontier is placed in the US would be a major change (Harrison and Schulz, 1989; Pollitt, 1987; 1991).

If that were to appear to be happening, however, we must not assume that doctors would simply content themselves with defending fixed positions. A more dynamic possibility is that they could counter-attack, taking over many management positions themselves. The involvement of clinicians, so earnestly sought by governments, could turn out to possess more than one aspect. No student of the history of the NHS should underestimate the capacity of doctors to adapt central initiatives and divert them locally, to their own ends. Doctor-managers may have a more diverse power-base then manager-managers, and be better able to resist central imperatives. Interestingly, 1991 witnessed the inaugural conference of the British Association of Medical Managers (Lyall, 1991).

Let us now set this possibility on one side. Assume, instead, that general managers do indeed secure increased control over what doctors do. We have suggested that what will then become crucial is the extent to which general managers can protect themselves from central interference and control. The general manager of the late 1980s was in part just an intelligent conduit for the flow of central directives and initiatives. If that flow really does diminish then the general manager of the mid 1990s could have much more room for manoeuvre. Our argument, however, has been that such a post-Fordist paradise though just conceivable, is unlikely. Political and economic pressures will most probably keep the stream running, and general managers harassed.

Beyond these specific power struggles there is the question of whether or not a broader cultural shift is taking place. Our own research suggested that among NHS staff, at least up to the end of 1988, there was little solid ground for any such assertion. Furthermore, we are sceptical of the claim (however common it may be in contemporary management texts) that top management can re-tool the culture of a large, complex organisation to suit its ends. We saw plenty of examples of new logos, newsletters, quality circles and so on, but whatever effects such devices may have they do not seem to alter the basic political appreciation of the situation held by many NHS staff. Managers continue to be seen as agents of the government in the way that doctors, nurses and other service-providers are not. The messages and proposals which come from managers are perceived accordingly – it is not that they are automatically disbelieved or regarded as worthless, but rather that they are 'screened' for possible contamination by central government's current political concerns. In a sentence, for most of the professional staff of the NHS general managers are not entirely trusted to speak and act in accordance with local rather than central interests. 'Management' is not a fully paid-up member of the NHS tribal club – it is seen (quite correctly in our view) as having divided loyalties.

Again, it is possible that this could change. The signs, however, are not particularly encouraging. *WfP* offers a vehicle for the further expansion of management influence, but equally *WfP* remains unpopular among NHS staff, as it does among the public at large. An expensive government advertising campaign has singularly failed to dent this resistance. 'The market' and the associated values of competitiveness and efficiency may have gained popularity in the public mind with respect to many other sectors during the 1980s, but seemingly not the NHS. The politician who was the most powerful advocate of applying a business model to the work of health authorities has been forced out of No 10. The Major cabinet seems more willing to acknowledge the 'specialness' of the public services, and to shift ministerial rhetoric from issues of efficiency to those of quality (Bevins, 1991; Timmins, 1991). Public satisfaction levels with NHS services may be slipping away from the very high levels achieved in previous decades, but what the public seems to want is a better NHS, not something completely different. The British public will tolerate a limited private sector in health care, but surveys also indicate that it discriminates between health services and most other services. It continues to resist any suggestion that most of its health care should be supplied through a market process.

References

Aaron, H. J and Schwartz, W. B. (1984) *The Painful Prescription: Rationing Hospital Care*. Washington D.C., Brookings Institution

Alford, R. R. (1975) *Health Care Politics*. Chicago, IU, University of Chicago Press

Allaire, Y. and Firsirotu, M. E. (1984) 'Theories of Organizational Culture', *Organization Studies*, **5** (3)

Allen, D. E. (1986) 'Trials and Tribulations of Fledgling DGMs', *Health Service Journal*, 10 April, 494

Allsop, J. (1984) *Health Policy and the National Health Service*. London, Longman

Alvesson, M. (1987) *Organization theory and technocratic consciousness: rationality, ideology and quality of work*. Berlin, de Gruyter

Andersen, T. F. and Mooney, G. (Eds.) *The Challenge of Medical Practice Variations*. London, Macmillan Press

Association of Community Health Councils for England and Wales (1988) *The Impact of General Management on the National Health Service: The Views of Community Health Councils*. London

Bachrach, P. and Baratz, M. S. (1962) 'The two faces of power', *American Political Science Review*, **56**, 947–52

Bachrach, P. and Baratz, M. S. (1970) *Power and Poverty: Theory and Practice*. London, Oxford University Press

Banyard, R. (1988a) 'How do UGMs Perform?', *Health Service Journal*, 21 July, 824–5

Banyard, R. (1988b) 'Management Mirrored', *Health Service Journal*, 28 July, 858–9

Banyard, R. (1988c) 'More Power to the Units', *Health Service Journal*, 4 August, 882–3

Banyard, R. (1988d) 'Watching the Revolution', *Health Service Journal*, 11 August, 916–17

Barbour, J. (1989) 'Notions of "success" in general management', *Health Services Management Research* **2** (1), 53–7

Bardsley, M. (1988) 'A Survey of the Use of Performance Indicator Packages in the NHS' in P. C. Berman (Ed.) *Management of Patient Care: Professionals a Managers in Search of New Alliances*. Utrecht, National Hospital Institute of the Netherlands

Barnard, K. and Harrison, S. (1986) 'Labour Relations in Health Services Management', *Social Science and Medicine*, **22** (11), 1213–28

Barnard, K., Lee, K., Mills, A., and Reynolds, J. (1979) *Towards a New Rationality: a Study of Planning in the NHS* (in four Volumes). University of Leeds, Nuffield Centre for Health Services Studies, Leeds

Barnard, K., Lee, K., Mills, A. and Reynolds J. (1980) 'NHS Planning: an

Assessment', *Hospital and Health Services Review*, **76** (8 & 9), 262–5, 301–4

Barrett, S. and McMahon, L. (1990) 'Public Management in Uncertainty: a Micro-political Perspective of the Health Service in the United Kingdom', *Policy and Politics*, **18** (4), 257–68

Bartlett, W. (1991) *Quasi-markets and contracts: a market and hierarchies perspective on NHS reform.* Bristol, School for Advanced Urban Studies, Decentralization and Quasi-Markets, Paper 3

Bate, P. (1984) 'The Impact of Organizational Culture on Approaches to Organizational Problem-Solving', *Organization Studies*, **5** (1)

Beardshaw, V., Hunter, D. J. and Taylor, R. (1990) *Local AIDS Policies: Planning and Policy Development for Health Promotion.* AIDS Programme Papers 6, London, Health Education Authority

Bevins, A. (1991) 'Tories' "must present compassionate image"', *The Independent*, 23 March, 6

Bloor, M. (1979) 'On the analysis of observational data: a discussion of the worth and uses of inducive techniques and respondent validation', *Sociology*, **12**, 545–52,

Boyd, K. M. (Ed.) (1979) *The Ethics of Resource Allocation in Health Care.* Edinburgh, University of Edinburgh Press

Brown, C. (1991) 'NHS internal market running out of money', *The Independent*, 11 July, 1

Brown, R. G. S. (1979) *Reorganising the National Health Service: A Case Study of Administrative Change.* Oxford, Blackwell and Martin Robertson

Brown, R. G. S., Griffin, S. and Haywood, S. C. (1975) *New Bottles: Old Wine?* Hull, University of Hull Institute for Health Studies

Buxton, M., Packwood, T. and Keen, J. (1989) *Resource Management: Process and Progress.* London, Department of Health

Buxton, M., Packwood, T. and Keen, J. (1991) *Final Report of the Brunel University Evaluation of Resource Management.* Uxbridge, Brunel University

Cameron, K. S. and Ettington, D. R. (1988) 'The Conceptual Foundations of Organizational Culture', in Smart, J. C. (Ed.), *Higher Education: Handbook of Theory and Research.* IV, 356–96. N.Y., Agathon Press.

Candlin, D. B. (1989) 'The Effective Plan', *Health Services Management Research*, **2** (2), 117–21

Caper, P. (1988) 'Solving the Medical Dilemma', *New England Journal of Medicine*, **318**, 1535–6

CASPE (1988) *How did we do? The use of performance indicators in the National Health Service.* London, CASPE Research

Castle, B. (1980) *The Castle Diaries 1974–76.* London, Weidenfeld and Nicolson

Cawson, A. (Ed.) (1985) *Organized Interests and the State: Studies in Meso-corporatism.* London, Sage

Chantler, C. (1988) *Guy's Hospital 1985–1988: a case study.* London, unpublished paper produced for the King's Fund International Fellowship series

Cochrane, A. (1972) *Effectiveness and Efficiency: Random Reflections on Health Services.* London, Nuffield Provincial Hospitals Trust

Coe, P. (1985) 'Teams with a Regional Accent', *Health and Social Service Journal*, October 3, 1232–3.

Committee of Enquiry into the Cost of the National Health Service (1956) (Chairman: Mr. C. W. Guillebaud), Report, Cmnd. 663, London, HMSO

Committee of Inquiry into Allegations of Ill-Treatment of Patients and Other Irregularities at Ely Hospital, Cardiff (1969). (Chairman: Mr Geofrey Howe), Report, London, HMSO

Committee of Inquiry into Normansfield Hospital (1978). (Chairman: Mr. M. D. Sherrard), Report, Cmnd. 7357, London, HMSO

Committee of Public Accounts (1990) *Financial Management in the National Health Service, 16th Report, Session 1989–90*. HC 102, London, HMSO

Committee on the Civil Service (1968). (Chairman: Lord Fulton), Report, Cmnd. 3638, London, HMSO

Confederation of Health Service Employees (1987) *Final Report: The Impact of General Managers in the NHS*. Banstead

Cook, R. (1990) *A fresh start for health*. London, Labour Party

Coombs, R and Cooper, D. (1990) *Accounting for Patients? Information Technology and the Implementation of the NHS White Paper*. PICT Policy Research Paper No. 10, Swindon, Economic and Social Research Council

Crossman, R. H. S. (1977) *The Diaries of a Cabinet Minister: Volume 3; Secretary of State for Social Services, 1968–70*. London, Hamish Hamilton and Jonathan Cape

Dahl, R. A. (1976) *Modern Political Analysis*. 3rd edn. Englewood Cliffs, N.J., Prentice Hall

Dalton, M. (1959) *Men Who Manage*. New York, Wiley

Day, P. and Klein, R. E. (1983) 'The Mobilisation of Consent versus the Management of Conflict: Decoding the Griffiths Report', *British Medical Journal*, **287**, 1813–15

Day, P. and Klein, R. (1987) *Accountabilities: Five Public Services*. London, Tavistock

Delamothe, T. (1990) 'Glasgow: City of Managerial Culture', *British Medical Journal*, **301**, 29 September, 654–6

Department of Health (1989b) *Medical audit, Working for Patients Working* Paper No. 6, London

Department of Health and Social Security (1970) *The Future Structure of the National Health Service*. (The Crossman Green Paper), London, HMSO

Department of Health and Social Security (1972a) *Management Arrangements for the Reorganised National Health Service*. London, HMSO

Department of Health and Social Security (1972b) *National Health Service Reorganisation: England*. Cmnd. 5055, London, HMSO

Department of Health and Social Security (1976) *Priorities for health and personal social services in England*. London, HMSO

Department of Health and Social Security (1982) 'NHS To Be Asked to Improve Accountability: Norman Fowler Announces New Moves and Regional Allocations', Press Release no. 82/14, 22 January

Department of Health and Social Security (1983) 'NHS Management Inquiry', Press Release no. 83/30, 3 February

Department of Health and Social Security (1984) *Health service management: implementation of the NHS management inquiry report*. HC(84)13, London, DHSS

Department of Health and Social Security and Welsh Office (1979) *Patients*

First: Consultative Paper on the Structure and Management of the National Health Service in England and Wales. London, HMSO

Department of Health, Welsh Office, Scottish Home and Health Department, and Northern Ireland Office (1989) *Working for Patients.* CM555, HMSO, London

Dopson, S. and Gabbay, J. (1987) 'What Should the DGM be Doing?', *Health Service Journal*, 14 May, 557

Dowding, K. (1992) *Rational Choice and Rational Power* (forthcoming)

Drucker, P. (1988) 'The Coming of New Organizations', *Harvard Business Review*, **66** (1), 45–53

East Anglian Regional Health Authority (1990) *Beyond the Windmill: Lessons from the Market Place* (revised edition) Cambridge

Elcock, H. and Haywood, S. (1980) *The Buck Stops Where? Accountability and Control in the National Health Service.* University of Hull, Hull, Institute for Health Studies

Elster, J. (1978) *Logic and Society: Contradictions and Possible Worlds.* Chicester, Wiley

Fairey, M. J., Condon, C., Darby, N., Donaldson, I., Kenny, D. and Wickings, I. (1975) *A Review of the Management of the Reorganised NHS.* London, Association of Chief Administrators of Health Authorities

Feldman, S. P. (1986) 'Management in Context: An Essay on the Relevance of Culture to the Understanding of Organizational Change', *Journal of Management Studies*, **23** (6), 587–607

Ferlie, E. and Pettigrew, A. M. (1988) 'AIDS: Responding to Rapid Change', *Health Service Journal*, 1 December, 1422–4

Ferlie, E. and Pettigrew, A. M. (1989) 'The Politics of Progress', *Health Service Journal*, 12 January, 44–6

Ferlie, E. and Pettigrew, A. M. (1990) 'Coping with change in the NHS: a frontline districts response to AIDS', *Journal of Social Policy*, **19**, (2), 191–220

Flynn, R. (1988) *Cutback Management in Health Services.* Department of Sociology and Anthropology, Salford, University of Salford

Forsyth, G. (1966) *Doctors and State Medicine: A Study of the British National Health Service.* London, Pitman Medical

Forte, P. G. L. (1986 *Decision-Making and Planning in a District Health Authority: A Review and a Case Study.* Working Paper no. 466, University of Leeds, School of Geography, Leeds

Fowler, N. (1982) Speech to Conservative Party Conference, 6 October, Issued in Conservative Party News Service Release no. 640/82

Frater, A. and Spiby, J. (1990) 'Groundwork for audit', *Health Service Journal*, 8th November, 1682

Freddi, G. (1989) 'Problems of organizational rationality in health systems: political controls and policy options' 1–27 in G. Freddi and J. W. Bjorkman (Eds.) *Controlling Medical Professionals the Comparative Politics of Health Governance.* London, Sage

Gabbay, J. and Stewart, R. (1987) 'Knowledge Needs Nurture', *Health Service Journal*, 23 July, 852

Gabbay, J. and Williams, D. (1987) 'Matching Managers with Members', *Health Service Journal*, 18 June, 706

Gabbay, J. and Williams, D. (1989) 'Community Physicians and General Managers: Experience and Expectations', *Journal of Management in Medicine*, **3** (3), 193

Gagliardi, P. (1986) 'The Creation and Change of Organizational Cultures: A Conceptual Framework', *Organization Studies*, **7** (2), 117–34

Glennerster, H. and Owens, P. (1986) *The Nursing Management Function After Griffiths: a Study in the North-West Thames Region*. London School of Economics and Political Science/North-West Thames RHA

Glennerster, H. and Owens, P. (1990) *Nursing in Conflict*. London, Macmillan

Glennerster, H., Korman, N. and Marslen-Wilson, F. (1983) 'Plans and Practice: the Participants' Views', *Public Administration*, **61** (3), 253–64

Green, S. (1975) 'Professional/Bureaucratic Conflict: the Case of the Medical Profession in the NHS', *Sociological Review*, **3** (1)

Griffiths, R. (1991) *Seven Years of Progress – General Management in the NHS*. Audit Commission Management Lectures No. 3, London, Audit Commission

Gunn, L. (1978) 'Why is Implementation so Difficult?' Management Services in Government, **33**, 169-176

Gunn, L. (1989) 'A Public Management Approach to the NHS, Health Services Management Research, 2 (1), 10–19

Habermas, J. (1971) *Towards a Rational Society*. London, Heinemann

Hallas, J. (1976) *CHCs in Action*. London, Nuffield Provincial Hospitals Trust

Ham, C. J. (1980) 'Community Health Council Participation in the NHS Planning System', *Social Policy and Administration*, **14** (3), 221–31

Ham, C. J. (1981) *Policy Making in the National Health Service*. London, Macmillan

Ham, C. (1985) *Health policy in Britain* (2nd edition). Basingstoke, Macmillan

Ham, C. J. (1986) *Managing Health Services: Health Authority Members in Search of a Role*. University of Bristol, Bristol, School for Advanced Urban Studies

Ham, C. (Ed.) (1988) *Health Care Variations: Assessing the Evidence*. Research Report 2, London, King's Fund Institute

Ham, C. (1991a) 'So far, so good?' *Health Service Journal*, 27 June, 22–3

Ham, C. (1991b) 'If it isn't hurting, it isn't working', *Marxism Today*, July, 14–17

Ham, C. and Hunter, D. J. (1988) *Managing Clinical Activity in the NHS*. Briefing Paper 8, London, King's Fund Institute

Hampton, J. R. (1983) 'The End of Clinical Freedom', *British Medical Journal*, **287**, 1237

Handy, C. (1985) *Gods of Management: the Changing Work of Organizations*. London, Souvenir Press

Handy, C. B. (1976) *Understanding Organizations*. Harmondsworth, Penguin

Hardy, B., Wistow, G. and Rhodes, R. A. W. (1990) 'Policy Networks and the Implementation of Community Care Policy for People with Mental Handicaps', *Journal of Social Policy*, **19** (2), 141–68

Hardy, C. (1986) 'Management in the NHS: Using Politics Effectively', *Public Policy and Adminstration*, **1**, 1–17

Harrison, S. (1981) 'The Politics of Health Manpower' in A. F. Long and G. Mercer (Eds.), *Manpower Planning in the National Health Service*. Farnborough, Gower Press.

Harrison, S. (1982) 'Consensus decision-making in the National Health Service: a review', *Journal of Management Studies*, **19** (4), 377–94

Harrison, S. (1988a) *Managing the National Health Service: Shifting the Frontier?*. London, Chapman and Hall

Harrison, S. (1988b), 'The Closed Shop and the National Health Service: A Case Study in Public Sector Labour Relations', *Journal of Social Policy*, **17** (1), 61–81

Harrison, S., Haywood, S. and Fussell, C. (1984) 'Problems and Solutions: the Perceptions of NHS Managers', *Hospital and Health Services Review*, **80** (4)

Harrison, S., Hunter, D. J., Marnoch, G. and Pollitt, C. J. (1988) 'Checkout on Griffiths: General Management in the NHS', *ESRC Newsletter*, **62**, 27–8

Harrison, S., Hunter, D. J., Marnoch, G. and Pollitt, C. (1989a) 'General Management and Medical Autonomy in the National Health Service', *Health Services Management Research* **2** (1), 38–46

Harrison, S. ; Hunter, D. J. and Pollitt, C. (1990) *The Dynamics of British Health Policy*. London, Unwin Hyman

Harrison, S., Hunter D. J., Pollitt, C. J. and Marnoch, G. (1989a) 'General Management and Medical Autonomy in the National Health Service', *Health Services Management Research*, **2** (1), 38–46

Harrison, S., Hunter, D. J., Marnoch, G. and Pollitt, C. (1989b) *The Impact of General Management in the National Health Service*. Milton Keynes, Open University

Harrison, S., Hunter, D. J., Pollitt, C. J. and Marnoch, G. (1989c) *General Management in the National Health Service: Before and After the White Paper*. Nuffield Institute Report No. 2, University of Leeds, Leeds, Nuffield Institute for Health Services Studies

Harrison, S., Hunter, D. J., Johnston, I and Wistow, G. (1989) *Competing for Health: A Commentary on the NHS Review*. Nuffield Institute Reports No. 1, University of Leeds, Leeds, Nuffield Institute for Health Services Studies

Harrison, S., Pohlman, C. E. and Mercer, G. (1984) *Concepts of Clinical Freedom Amongst English Physicians*. Paper Presented by EAPHSS Conference on Clinical Autonomy, King's Fund Centre, 8 June

Harrison, S. and Schulz, R. I. (1988) 'Impact of the Griffiths Reforms of National Health Service Management: the Views of Psychiatrists', *Health Services Management Research*, **1** (3), 127–34

Harrison, S. and Schulz, R. I. (1989) 'Clinical autonomy in the United Kingdom and the United States: contrasts and convergence', 198–209 in G. Freddi and J. W. Bjorkman (Eds.) *Controlling medical professionals; the comparative politics of health governance*. London, Sage

Haywood, S. C. (1977) *Decision Making in the New NHS: Consensus or Constipation*. King's Fund Project Paper no. 17, London

Haywood, S. C. (1979) 'Team Management in the NHS: What is it all About?', *Health and Social Service Journal*, Centre 8 Paper, 5 October

Haywood, S. C. (1983), *District Health Authorities in Action*. University of Birmingham, Research Report no. 19, Birmingham, Health Services Management Centre.

Haywood, S. C. and Alaszewski, A. (1980) *Crisis in the Health Service: the Politics of Management*. London, Croom Helm

Haywood, S. C., Alaszewski, A., Elcock, H. J., James, T. L. and Law, E. (1979) *The Curate's Egg . . . Good in Parts: Senior Officer Reflections on the NHS*. University of Hull, Hull, Institute for Health Studies

Haywood, S. and Hunter, D. J. (1982) 'Consultative processes in health policy in the United Kingdom: a view from the 'centre', *Public Administration*, **60** (2), 143–62

Haywood, S. C., Monks, A., and Webster, D. (1989) *Efficiency in the National Health Service*. Birmingham, University of Birmingham Health Services Management Centre

Haywood, S. C. and Ranadé, W. (1985) *District Health Authorities in Action: Two Years On*. University of Birmingham, Birmingham, Health Services Management Centre

Health Service Journal (1991) 'Doubts persist on the reforms', 11th July, 17

Heclo, H. (1975) *Modern Social Politics in Britain and Sweden*. London, Yale University Press

Heller, T. (1979) *Restructuring the Health Service*. London, Croom Helm

Henley, D., Holtham, C., Likierman, A. and Perrin, J. R. (1986) *Public Sector Accounting and Financial Control*. Wokingham, Van Nostrand Reinhold/CIPFA

Herzlinger, R. E. (1989) 'The Failed Revolution in Health Care . . . the Role of Management', *Harvard Business Review*, March-April, 95-103

Hinings, C. R., Hickson, D. J., Pennings, J. M. and Schneck, R. E. (1971) 'Structured Conditions of Intraorganisational Power', *Administrative Science Quarterly*, **16** (2), June

Hoggett, P. (1990) *Modernisation, Political Strategy and the Welfare State: an Organizational Perspective*. Studies in Decentralization and Quasi-Markets No. 2, Bristol, School for Advanced Urban Studies

Holland, W. W. (Ed.) (1983) *Evaluation of Health Care*. Oxford, Oxford University Press

Hood, C. (19??) 'A Public Management For All Seasons?', *Public Administration*, **69** (1), 3–19

Hughes, D. (1989) 'Paper and People: the Work of the Casualty Reception Clerk', *Sociology of Health and Illness*, **11** (4), 382–408

Hunter, D. J. (1979) 'Practice: Decisions and Resources in the National Health Service (Scotland)' in K. M. Boyd (Eds.) *The Ethics of Resource Allocation in Health Care*. Edinburgh, Edinburgh University Press

Hunter, D. J. (1980) *Coping with Uncertainty*. Letchworth, Research Studies Press

Hunter, D. J. (1982) 'Organising for Health: The National Health Service in the United Kingdom', *Journal of Public Policy*, **2**, 263–300

Hunter, D. J. (1984a) 'Managing Health Care', *Social Policy and Administration*, **18** (1), 41–67

Hunter, D. J. (1984b) 'NHS Management: is Griffiths the Last Quick Fix?', *Public Administration*, **62** (1), 91–4

Hunter, D. J. (1986) *Managing the NHS in Scotland: Review and Assessment of Research Issues*. Edinburgh, Scottish Home and Health Department

Hunter, D. J. (1988) 'The Impact of Research on Restructuring the British National Health Service', *The Journal of Health Administration Education*, **6** (3), 537–53

Hunter, D. J. (1990) 'Managing the Cracks: Managing Development for Health Care Interfaces', *The International Journal of Health Planning and Managment*, **5** (1), 7–14

Hunter, D. J. (1992) 'Doctors as Managers: Gamekeepers Turned Poachers?', *Social Science and Medicine*, **33**

Hunter, D. J. and Wistow, G. (1987) *Community Care in Britain: Variations on a Theme*. London, King Edward's Hospital Fund for London

Hunter, D. J. and Williamson, P. (1991) 'Comparisons and Contrats between Scotland and England', *Health Services Management*, **87** (4), 166–70

Illich, I. (1977) *Limits to Medicine*. Harmondsworth, Penguin

Illich, I.*et al.*(1977) *Disabling Professions*. London, Marion Boyars

Illsley, R. (1980) *Professional or Public Health? Sociology in Health and Medicine*. London, Nuffield Provincial Hospitals Trust

Institute of Health Service Administrators (1984) 'Letter to the Secretary of State for Social Services' in Social Services Committee, First Report 1983–84: Griffiths NHS Management Inquiry Report, HC 209, House of Commons/HMSO, London

Jaques, E. (Ed.) (1978) *Health Services*. London, Heinemann

Jenkins, L., Bardsley, M., Coles, J., Wickings, I., and Leow, H. (1987) *Use and Validity of NHS Performance Indicators . . . A National Survey*. London, CASPE Research/King's Fund

Jenkins, L., Bardsley, M., Coles, J. and Wickings, I. (1988) *How Did We Do? The Use of Performance Indicators in the National Health Service*. London, CASPE Research

Johnston, R. and Lawrence, P. R. (1988) 'Beyond vertical integration . . . the rise of the value-adding partnership' *Harvard Business Review*, July/August, 94–101

Joint Working Party (1967). (Chairman: Mr. G. P. E. Howard) *The Shape of Hospital Management in 1980?* London, King Edward's Hospital Fund for London

Jones, T. and Prowle, M. (1984) *Health Service Finance: an Introduction* (2nd edn). London Certified Accountants Educational Trust

Keynes, J. M. (1936) *The General Theory of Employment, Interest and Money*. London, Macmillan

King's Fund Institute (1988) *Health finance: assessing the options*. Briefing Paper 4, London, King's Fund Institute

Klein, R. (1989) 'Normansfield: Vacuum of Management in the NHS', *British Medical Journal*, **ii**, 1802–4

Klein, R. E. (1984) 'Who Makes Decisions in the NHS?', *British Medical Journal*, **288** (2)

Klein, R. (1989) *The Politics of the NHS* (2nd edn). London, Longman

Klein, R. E and Lewis, J. (1976) *The Politics of Consumer Representation*. London, Centre for Studies in Social Policy

Kogan, M., Goodwin, B., Henkel, M., Korman, N., Packwood, T., Bush, A., Hoyes, V., Ash, L. and Tester J. (1978) *The Working of the National Health Service*.Royal Commission of the National Health Service, Research Paper no. 1., London, HMSO

Korman, N. and Glennerster, H. (1990) *Hospital Closure*. Milton Keynes, Open University Press

Kotter, J. P. (1982) *The General Managers*. New York, Free Press

Lee, K. and Mills, A. (1982) *Policy-Making and Planning in the Health Sector.* London, Croom Helm

Lee, R. and Lawrence, P. (1985) *Organizational Behaviour: Politics at Work.* London, Hutchinson.

Levitt, R. (1979) *The Regoranised National Health Service* (2nd edn). London, Croom Helm

Levitt, R and Wall, A. (1984) *The Reorganised National Health Service.* London, Croom Helm

Liddell, A. (1988) 'General management in a district health authority' in Barbara Stocking (Ed.), *In dreams begin responsibility: a tribute to Tom Evans.* London, King Edward's Hospital Fund for London

Liddell, A. and Parston, G. (1990) 'How the market crashed', *Health Service Journal,* 17th May, 730–2

Light, D. and Levine, S. (1989) 'The Changing Character of the Medical Profession: a Theoretical Overview', *The Milbank Quarterly,* **66**, Supplement 2

Lindblom, C. E. (1959) 'The Science of Muddling Through', *Public Administration Review,* **19** (3), 79–88

Lindblom, C. E. (1979 'Still Muddling, Not Yet Through', *Public Administration Review,* **39** (6), 517–26

Linstead, D. (1984) 'The Realities of Human Resourcing: a Case Study which Questions the Utility of Rational Manpower Planning Models in Health Care', *Health Services Manpower Review,* **10** (3), 9–11

Lipietz, A. (1987) *Mirages and miracles.* London, Verso

Lipsky, M. (1980) *Street-Level Bureaucracy.* New York, Russell Sage Foundation

Lukes, S. (1974) *Power: A Radical View.* London, Macmillan

Lyall, J. (1991) 'Donning a management hat with aplomb', *Health Service Journal,* 20 June, 14–15

MacLachlan, R. (1990) 'Where patients become judges of success', *Health Service Journal,* 12 July, 1026–7

McKee, L. (1988) 'Conflicts and Context in Managing the Closure of a Large Psychiatric Hospital', *Bulletin of the Royal College of Psychiatrists,* **12** (8), 310–19

McKee L. and Pettigrew, A. M. (1988) 'Managing Major Change', *Health Service Journal,* 17 November, 1358–60

McKee, L. and Pettigrew, A. M. (1989) 'Hospitals do not hurry', *Health Service Journal,* 26 January, 102–4

McKeganey, N. P. and Bloor, M. (1981) 'On the retrieval of sociological descriptions: respondent validations and the critical care of ethnomethodology', *International Journal of Sociology and Social Policy,* **1** (3), 58–69

Marnoch, G., Harrison, S., Hunter, D. J. and Pollitt, C. J. (1989) 'After the Culture Shock', *Health Services Journal,* 7 December, 1500–1

May, A. (1991) 'Turning round the aircraft carrier', *Health Service Journal,* 20 June, 14

Meek, V. L. (1988) 'Organizational culture: origins and weaknesses', *Organization Studies,* **9** (4), 453–73

Millar, B. (1990a) 'Up in the air after a smooth take off', *Health Service Journal,* 26 July, 1105

Millar, B. (1990b) 'Calling all farmers and business gurus', *Health Service Journal*, 16 August, 1207

Millar, B. (1990c) 'Emerging from the golden chrysalis', *Health Service Journal*, 17 May, 1720–1.

Mills, I. (1987) 'Regional Realism: Reaping Rewards', *Health Service Journal*, 23 April, 470–1

Ministry of Health and Department of Health for Scotland (1944) *A National Health Service*. Cmnd. 6502, London, HMSO

Ministry of Health and Scottish Home and Health Department (1966). (Chairman: Mr. Brian Salmon) *Report of the Committee on Senior Nursing Staff Structure*. London, HMSO

Mintzberg, H. (1973) *The Nature of Managerial Work*. Englewood Cliffs, N.J., Prentice Hall

Mooney, G. and Loft, A. (1989) 'Clinical decision making and health care policy: what is the link?' *Health Policy*, **11**, 19–25

Mulgen, G. (1988) 'The power of the weak', *Marxism Today*, December, 24–31

National Health Service Management Inquiry (1983) *Report ('The Griffiths Report')*. London, Department of Health and Social Security

NHS Management Executive (1989) *Quality*. Chief Executive's letter to Regional and District General Managers, EL(89)/MB/117

Naylor, W. M. (1971) *Organisation and Management of a Unified Health Service: Organisation of Area Health Services*. London, Institute of Health Service Administrators

Notman, M., Howe, K. R., Rittenberg, W., Bridgham, R., Holmes, M. M and Rovner, D. R. (1987) 'Social Policy and Professional Self-interest: Physician Responses to DRGs', *Social Science and Medicine*, **25**, 1259–67

O'Sullivan, J. (1990) 'Leeds disunited over "Jimmy's" opt-out plan', *The Independent*, 7 July, 3

O'Sullivan, J. (1991) 'GPs freedom to spend budgets may be limited', *The Independent*, 8 June, 3

Olsen (1971)

Owens, P. and Glennerster, H. (1988) *The Nursing Management Function After Griffiths: A Study in the North-West Thames Region: A Second Interim Report*. London School of Economics and Political Science/North-West Thames RHA

Packwood, T. ; Keen, J. and Buxton, M. (1991) *Hospitals in Transition: the Resource Management Experiment*. Milton Keynes, Open University Press

Pater, J. E. (1981) *The Making of the National Health Service*. London, King Edward's Hospital Fund

Petchey, R. (1986) 'The Griffiths Reorganisation of the National Health Service: Fowlerism by Stealth?', *Critical Social Policy*, **6** (2), 87–101

Peters T. J. and Waterman, R. H. (1982) *In Search of Excellence*. New York, Harper and Row

Pettigrew, A. M. (1973) *The Politics of Organizational Decisionmaking*. London, Tavistock

Pettigrew, A. M., McKee, L. and Ferlie, E. (1988) 'Wind of Change Blows through NHS Research', *Health Service Journal*, 3 November, 1296–8

Pettigrew, A., McKee, L. and Ferlie, E. (1989a) 'Hints on How to Ring the Changes', *Health Service Journal*, 16 February, 200–2

Pettigrew, A., McKee, L. and Ferlie, E. (1989b) 'Managing Strategic Service Change in the NHS', *Health Services Management Research*, 2 (1), 20–31

Pfeffer, J. (1978) *Organizational Design*. Arlington Heights, IU, AHM Publishing Corporation.

Pfeffer, J. (1981) *Power in Organizations*. Pitman, Marshfield, Mass

Pfeffer, J. and Salancik, G. R. (1978) *The External Control of Organizations: A Resource Dependence Perspective*. New York, Harper and Row

Pindar, K. (1986) 'The Visible Persuaders', *Health Care Management*, 1 (1) 3–9

Pohlman, C. E. (1985) *Clinical Autonomy and Health Service Management*. Unpublished M. A. Dissertation, University of Wisconsin-Madison

Pollitt, C. (1986) 'Beyond the managerial model: performance assessment in government and the public services', *Financial Accountability and Management*, 2 (3), 155–70

Pollitt, C (1987) 'Capturing quality? The quality issue in British and American health policies', *Journal of Public Policy*, 7 (1), 71–92

Pollitt, C. (1990a) *Managerialism and the Public Services: the Anglo-American Experience*. Oxford, Blackwell

Pollitt, C. (1990b) 'Doing business in the temple? Managers and quality assurance in the public services', *Public Administration*, 68 (4)

Pollitt, C. (1991) *The politics of medical quality: auditing doctors in the UK and the USA*. Paper presented to the annual conference of the Political Studies Association, Lancaster, 15–17 April

Pollitt, C. J., Harrison, S., Hunter, D. J., and Marnoch, G. (1988) 'The Reluctant Managers: Clinicians and Budgets in the NHS', *Financial Accountability and Management*, 4 (3), 213–34

Pollitt, C. J., Harrison, S., Hunter, D. J. and Marnoch, G. (1989) *Improving Organizational Performance: Mirage and Reality in Health Service Management*. Occasional Paper no. 3, Brussels, European Group of Public Administration

Pollitt, C. J., Harrison, S., Hunter, D. J. and Marnoch, G. (1990) 'No hiding place: on the discomforts of researching the contemporary policy process', *Journal of Social Policy*, 19 (2), 169–90

Polsby, N. W. (1980) *Community Power and Political Theory: A Further Look at Problems of Evidence and Inference* (2nd edn), New Haven CT, Yale University Press

Powell, J. E. (1966) *Medicine and Politics*. London, Pitman Medical

Rathwell, T. A. (1987) *Strategic Planning in the Health Sector*. London, Croom Helm

Rayner, Lord (1984) *The Unfinished Agenda* (Stamp Memorial Lecture). University of London

Rhodes, R. A. W. (1986) 'Corporate Bias in Central-Local Relations: A Case Study of the Consultative Council on Local Government Finance', *Policy and Politics*, 14 (2), 221–45

Rivlin, A. (1971) 'Obstacles to Social Progress: Why Can't We Get Things Done', *Washington Post*, 22 July

Robinson, J. and Strong, P. (1987) *Professional Nursing Advice After Griffiths: An Interim Report*. Coventry, Warks, University of Warwick Nursing Policy Studies Centre

Robinson, J., Strong, P. and Elkan, R. (1989) *Griffiths and the Nurses: a*

National Survey of CNAs. Nursing Policy Studies no. 4, Coventry, Warks, University of Warwick Nursing Policy Studies Centre

Royal College of Physicians (1989) *Medical audit: a first report: what, why and how?*, London, RCP, March.

Royal College of Surgeons (1989) *Guidelines to clinical audit in surgical practice*. RCS, London, March

Rowbottom, R.*et al*.(1973) *Hospital Organisation*. Heinemann, London

Sabatier, P. A. (1986) 'What can we learn from implementation research?', 313–25 in Franz-Xaver Kaufman, Giandomedico Majone and Vincent Ostrom, *Guidance, control and evaluation in the public sector*, Berlin, de Gruyter

Sartori, G. (1987) *The Theory of Democracy Re-visited: part one: The Contemporary Debate*. New Jersey, Chatham House

Scarfe, J. (1987) *The Greenwich Project*. (3rd year undergraduate project), Norwich, University of East Anglia, School of Economic and Social Studies

Schmitter, P. C. (1974) 'Still the Century of Corporatism?', *Review of Politics*, **36**, 85–131

Schulz, R. I and Harrison, S. (1983) *Teams and Top Managers in the NHS: A Survey and a Strategy*. King's Fund Project Paper no. 41, London

Scottish Health Services Council (1966). (Chairman: Mr. W. M. Farquharson-Lang) Administrative Practice of Hospital Boards in Scotland, Edinburgh, HMSO

Scrivens, E. (1988a) 'The Management of Clinicians in the Hospitals of the English National Health Service' in P. C. Berman (Ed.) *Management of Patient Care: Professionals and Managers in Search of New Alliances*. Utrecht, National Hospitals Institute of the Netherlands

Scrivens, E. (1988b) 'The Management of Clinicians in the National Health Service', *Social Policy and Administration*, **22** (1), 22–34

Scrivens, E. (1988c) 'Doctors and Managers: Never the Twain Shall Meet?' *British Medical Journal*, **296**, 1754–5

Siedentopf, H. (1982) 'Introduction: government performance and administrative reform', ixxv in Gerald E. Caiden and Heinrich Siedentopf (Eds.), *Strategies for administrative reform*. Lexington Mass., Lexington Books

Smith, P. (1987) 'The new-style manager gets wheels turning', *Health Service Journal*, 21 May, 584–5

Smith, R. (1990) 'Enter the men from the Audit Commission', *British Medical Journal*, **301**, 1269–72, 1st December

Social Services Committee (1984) *First Report*. Session 1983–84: Griffiths NHS Management Inquiry Report, HC 209, London, House of Commons/HMSO

Stephenson, T. E. (1985) *Management: A Political Activity*. London, Macmillan

Stewart, R. (1989) 'Pressures and Constraints on General Management', *Health Services Management Research*, **2** (1), 32–7

Stewart, Rosemary and Dopson, S. (1987) *DGMs and region*. Templeton College series on District General Managers No. 6, National Health Service Training Authority

Stewart, R., Smith, P., Blake, J. and Wingate, P. (1980) *The District Administrator in the National Health Service*. London, King's Fund

Stocking, B. (1985) *Initiative and Inertia: Case Studies in the NHS*. London, Nuffield Provincial Hospitals Trust

Storey, J. (1990) 'Human resource management in the public sector', *Public Money and Management*, **9** (3), 19–24.

Strong, P. and Robinson, J. (1988a) *New Model Management: Griffiths and the NHS*. Nursing Policy Studies no. 3, Coventry, Warks, University of Warwick Nursing Policy Studies Centre

Strong, P. and Robinson, J. (1988b), 'Warts and All', *Nursing Times*, **84**, (39), 53–4

Strong, P. and Robinson J. (1990), *The NHS Under New Management*. Milton Keynes, Open University Press

Symes, D. (1988) 'Professionals and Managers . . . Report on a Survey of Current Practice', Unpublished

Thompson, D. J. C. (1986) *Coalition and Decision-Making Within Health Districts*. Research Report no. 23, University of Birmingham, Birmingham Health Services Management Centre

Thompson, D. (1990) 'Organisation Studies: Time for Change', *Health Services Management*, **86** (6), 270–2

Thompson, F. J. (1981) *Health Policy and the Bureaucracy: Politics and Implementation*. Cambridge, Massachusetts, The MIT Press

Timmins, N. (1985). 'And May the Best Man Be Vetoed', *The Times*, 21 January

Timmins, N. (1991) 'Major spells out his plan for the decade' *The Independent*, 23 July, 1

Timmins, N. and Jones, J. (1991) 'Labour dismisses charter as "£8M fraud"' *The Independent*, 24 July, 5

Tomlin, Z. (1990) 'Hurdles on the path to medical audit', *Health Service Journal*, 26 July, 1104

Tomlin, Z. (1991a) 'First faltering steps towards an outcome', *Health Service Journal*, 18 July, 13

Tomlin, Z. (1991b) 'The placid watchdog has learned to bite', *Health Service Journal*, 11 July, 13

Turnor, B. A. (Ed.) (1990) *Organizational Symbolism*. New York, de Gruyter

Watkin, B. (1975) *Documents on Health and Social Services: 1834 to the Present Day*. London, Methuen

Webb, A., Wistow, G. and Hardy, B. (1986) *Structuring Local Policy Environments: Central-Local Relations in the Health and Personal Social Services: Final Report to the ESRC*. Loughborough, Centre for Research in Social Policy

Weiner, S. L., Maxwell, J. H., Sapolsky, H. M., Dunn, D. L and Hsiao, W. C. (1987) 'Economic Incentives and Organisational Realities: Managing Hospitals Under DRGs', *The Millbank Quarterly*, **65**, 463–87

Williamson, P. (1990) *General Management in the Scottish Health Service*. Department of Community Medicine, Aberdeen, University of Aberdeen

Wiseman, C. (1979) 'Strategic Planning in the Scottish Health Service . . . A Mixed-Scanning Approach', *Long Range Planning*, **12** (2), 103–13

Zuboff, S. (1988) *In the age of the smart machine: the future of work and power*. Oxford, Heinemann

Index